The Red Pulpit

A journey into psychosis
– and out again

Robert Morrison

Lee Green Press

Copyright © Robert Morrison

The right of author to be identified as the author of this work has been asserted by him in accordance with the Copyright, Designs and Patent Act 1988.

All rights reserved. No part of this work may be published or otherwise circulated in any form without the express permission of the publisher.

ISBN 978-1-84327-940-2

Cover design:; Electric Book
First published in Great Britain 2013.

Lee Green Press

Lee Green Press is the imprint of Lee Green Community Centre
3 Leegate, Lee
London SE12 8SS, UK
Registered charity 1141238

To Lynn

Rob Morrison comes from London where he doesn't live with his family and his four dogs. He almost certainly didn't go to Cambridge, isn't anything special and hasn't 'done' Australia. He expects to never drive, and to continue eating at his local curry parlour; his waistband yet again is emerging. Gods have preached and yelled at Rob from their red pulpit and promised this and that. He eventually doused their fanatical flame and breathed fire himself.

PREFACE

Psychosis sells. It's in the industrial income bracket. That fine line between sanity and madness becomes marketable as individualism. Today a lack of spontaneous creativity seems a guarantee of integrity. Incredulity! Damien Hurst is E.E.Cummings is suicidal British actor Robert Carlisle. It's all interchangeable. I'll have Belinda Carlisle, singer of pretty pop songs and simply beautiful from whatever angle the psychotic, hair-fluffed art inspector will distinguish between her innocent solo image and the Go-Go's.

To be psychotic in the modern world is to guarantee the old genius of King Lear, even though he was creatively undistinguished and rescued by the love and faithfulness of the daughter he had once impetuously banished. Real "genius" is emphatically more possible without psychosis. The following pages have been titled 'the red pulpit' because it is I who have suffered and met that fate. I can be wackily complex and a flamboyant dresser, but I challenge anybody brave enough to stand there and call it a celebration of wild parties, wine, women and song - or art. I have changed for the better, but there was no plan to it, and to overcome it was like an ant climbing Mount Everest, at least twice. Let those illusions rest with the ad-man. In this account and not for the first time, I am aware of controversial beliefs and symptoms that were no more than a disfigurement of reality in the broadest sense. I hope this doesn't spoil but rather enhance the benefit a sufferer or otherwise may get from reading this account. The only justice I can do you is to try and tell it like it is.

Robert Morrison

THE GOOD

1

This is the story of a dark night. This is the account of inertia in an ever-expanding universe. This is the document of wrong prevailing over healthy expectation. In my life I tilled the soil, I fed the livestock and I fetched water from the well. I was a slave to the crowing call for lunch and I gobbled passionately like a scavenging pigeon when it came, dependant on the respectful giving of a few children. I never won a general election or bagged prize scalps on Pop Idol, and by the end I never cared much for dreams.

I read somewhere once that biographies were better than autobiographies because they were written in the third person. I suppose they meant that writing an autobiography could be a bit like an inadequate talking about himself over dinner where an audience could only ascertain an unsubtle bias of trumpet-blowing and gesticulation. However, in his defence the biographer would only choose the story of a media-hero to slap on a publisher's desk because the blithering idiot wouldn't want to spend twenty pounds on anything else. Thus the person who sets out to write about an unglamorous second-cousin to Art Garfunkel (if he's lucky) such as me, can only be me. Besides, when I'm at dinner parties, my trumpet is firmly lost among the worn Glenn Miller LP's in the broom-cupboard under the stairs, as I strain to analyze syntax from my deftly concealed quotations manual between my knees. Recognize him? If you were a publishing agent in this vaunted company would you be 'blithering' enough to put up with the incessant wittering of a failed writer with all the finesse of a DC10? If you're like-minded, to research the meaty bits of this book, you could catch some video footage of the

Remedial Book Programme or wait for the edited highlights of Crimewatch instead of drowsily snuggling up to a hot-water bottle and a 'good' book about an outstanding journey of a lifetime. That could not replace the sadness and pain of this document's honest and truthful lifetime's journey. If you are plucky enough to mention my book at our gathering you too may have given up the ghost by page five and bluffed your way through with your equally lost rivals in time for coffee and Trivial Pursuits. I'd do it. Thus, I cannot open my written repertoire with a performance of the Grieg piano concerto on the trumpet but just be satisfied that the book does justice to me, fairly. Mission accomplished. If anyone is interested in reading the rest, my name is Robert and I tilled the soil, fed the livestock and fetched water from the well, and if I am less than loquacious I still feel free to talk about myself in the first person and that is why I have chosen to 'have a go' and write an autobiography.

The success of biographies stems from the subject being written about and less from the writer of the subject. In crude terms the readership wants to know the subject a little more personally than the author and this is understandable. In an autobiography the subject ought to be judged as a writer and his cards sent for if he is not adequate and didn't send for the biographer in the first place. This is why Rio Ferdinand never wrote an autobiography. Thus if I'm honest I have to fulfill the dubious duality of being both a decent enough writer about a decent enough subject to win my readership over. My life should involve a cartload of anecdotes, sharp analysis and subtle innuendo, one might think. A single incident that made waves should not engulf the life-story for they seldom make up the whole individual. Yes, we should know what the subject did privately, but not without cancelling the light upon who that person really is. A biography of Gerald Ratner would be stale if after three years one picked up a biography and it read about a quote documenting a "bunch of crap". That's not all he was surely? His company was ruined by hostile media-coverage and the mass-reading public buying into the hysteria of one, albeit supersonic faux-pas. That is what should feature heavily in a book about this public figure, not that he let his pants down and did an ocean-wide moony.

Human behaviour after-all, is shared behaviour and we are all capable of doing the same worthy and worthless things. However behaviour can often be no more than an outward expression of the inner consciousness, but sometimes we forget this and in doing so don't understand our own reasons for such actions. Does anyone really care about being honest when we are presented with food and drink we know nothing about in a restaurant? No. Our answer is always the same. If the wine tastes like Tizer, it's always remarkable vintage and if the steak's a bit tough, we forget that most of us have not much more culinary expertise than a plate of egg and chips.

The same is true of the subject of a biography who will probably be as lost in a restaurant or supermarket as you and me. But in establishing our similarities why does it make it necessary to relate our own shared, innate, human response in words. The reason is because people either past or present are unique. It is my belief that although we stem from the same life force I will never be a Peter Ustinov or a Jim Davidson, but depending on how life treats me, I have the potential in me to be far more or far less than these men that fate will allow. It is that kind of individual essence that I want people to read about and that which we really have and that which we really are. That's who I am and who I can make the subject of his own gripping autobiography. He who pisses in the well has no ego.

I enrolled on a writing course once and one of the three

lessons I attended was about how best to describe the passage of time in an account. The group members agreed on the whole that time should unfold from where the plot is at its height. In other words the plot should zap all around like Mick Jagger. This has a reputation for being contemporary wisdom, although is it? In the movie 'Shine', the child-piano-prodigy, David Helfgott begins by hammering on the glass of an Australian pub obviously distressed and for the next hour the audience is told how he arrived in such a mess. Was this so absolutely necessary? It may be a great film but starting it near the end spoils some of the surprise as from the outset we know that David Helfgott is going to crack up. And that's contemporary wisdom.

However, not to sound like a door-to-door salesman, I write for passion, not fashion. I am as green as a small water lily in a big pond as you can see, but the standard of British writers some of whom begin their stories halfway through, do little to impress me, even though they probably consider me fair-game for the five-ninety-nine I have spent on Posh Spice's top tips on rare foot complaints, to prove they are really necessary to the British literary scene.

In this life-story the format will be as it comes which may be confusing but certainly fresh from the memory to the page. The pivotal moment of my account may ambush without pre-warning or it may not. It is possible that I still await my pivotal moment.

I will approach this format at the beginning. I am Robert Arthur Morrison and my initials spell RAM that stands for many acronyms beside the Royal Academy of Music for which they were selected. The middle name I counted as an embarrassing expletive, especially when it lay dormant in the school register, waiting for one of my more curious mortal enemies to pounce on. In actual fact school chums who did stumble across my oft-mumbled secret were completely unruffled. It was always me who was sensitive. Mark Kingsley Hunt and Andrew Alfonso Thompson had much more to squeal about. Andy the Unflappable probably didn't deserve Ian either, and his acronym surely enough was AIL so I wasn't alone in my melancholia. Paul kindly mentioned, perhaps too kindly that it was cool to be called Arthur, because "look at Arthur Fonzarelli out of Happy Days". However it was clear to me that there were no parallels at all to be drawn from myself and the Fonz. On his planet the female species were driven crazy by boys in leather and on my planet if you called "Hey!" to anyone they would shout "Hey!" back. If I tried charm that was no use either. Most girls would spit their gum to the ground, vacantly stare past me and say "Hey?" It should have been highlighted at a young age that I was to young girls what Richie Cunningham was to cardigans. Out of the two of us, I was the bigger dick. Although I was stuck with Arthur, I took no stick at all because the early eighties saw a plethora of lovable 'Arfurs" emerge as the press called them. Since every schoolboy in my age group was hooked on Minder, I had no reason to look back, at least, not in anger.

And on the subject of padding, my other two names ought to fit the impression of who I am, but I don't suppose Robert or Morrison give an accurate assessment. The whole name suggests I could come from anywhere in the British Isles excusing Ireland. So whom am I patriotic towards? To who do I sincerely belong? One is probably completely disinterested by this, and it's not even page five, but I have reason to announce that I belong to the English, the nation being swallowed up by an ever-growing identity crisis. Many sophisticates argue that today Englishness is presently hard to define and yet deny that it was their own ignorance of the real world that allowed this state of affairs to germinate. Who would argue that with so many nationalities and identities living under British skies that to define an Englishman would now be complex? However with the situation being so bad I would counter that it is even more difficult to define an Englishman in this country if he happens to be an Englishman! When ruminating over the Englishness question I am often gently brought back to that canny movie, "Sleuth" by playwright Antony Shaffer, which unlocks the key to being English, strangely through the words of Michael Caine's character who is humiliated by a very blue-blooded Laurence Olivier. In Olivier's game Caine is humiliated to a whimpering wife-snatcher, imploring for his own life not to be taken by the adversarial husband. Olivier shows no mercy. Caine is of Italian descent and cannot graduate to the English society to which he belongs. And then Caine clinches the game he is about to lose, by claiming he belongs to a "fair play and sense of humour England " and this for me depicts my Englishness apart from other peoples living on this planet. There are Englishmen who will no doubt disagree with me upon this interpretation but generally they have no more feelings of belonging somewhere than Tommy Docherty. I propose that most English people will agree with me. Perhaps it is no mystery that as an island we are cut off from the Germans and enjoy flourishing humour and fair-play! Yikes! Although my home has always been in England, the cities up and down the country and those in which I have lived do not necessarily imply a common bond of heritage. England can surely be as diverse as it is divided. The western counties and the eastern counties speak the same tongue but are no nearer to a common identity than North or South Korea. If Alan Whicker campaigned for Truro to be twinned with Lowestoft, it would probably be met with approval on both sides of the M11, but in local government, east doesn't mean the East End but the Soviet Union. There is a lot more to east meets west than frozen turkeys and cider apples. Why do English authorities continue to forage links with a commonwealth of nations while keeping its regional traditions foreign to its inhabitants.

London moreover, has more identities than telephone wires and yet finally the boundaries are the same for him as would be for a Dorsetshire weaver with each citizen currently dependant on a handful of friends that cut him off from somebody else's handful of friends. Is that not life I hear you ask, but perhaps London is the odd man out because here life never slows down, whereas maybe other townships pace a more even pattern. Here, big city life defines what life is. It is difficult to say if that's good. Some prefer the hectic open highway to the sedate and safe avenues of strawberry sponge recipes. The world here has over eight million creatures but occasionally through phone calls, only a couple of trusted friends can help him believe in the decency of his habitat again. In London, with so many inhabitants, most of us subconsciously switch off from our love affair with the real Big Brother except the girl in the packed train carriage whose mobile is definitely switched on.

London is a big city in England. However in the rear view mirrors of politicians it has to have become England in the last few decades, principally because, such is democracy in this country that a politician can quite effectively sell himself here and still be elected somewhere in the North East, helping himself to another five year stint in Number Ten with a terrifying propensity to do 'the right thing' with Iraq. Does he only ever show up in Newcastle in emergencies? No. Why should he? However in defence of our custodians at least they can say they might have been to the north which is more than I can say for the media. The press is London, and that's why it is full of bastards: I'll leave the reader to decide which one is 'it'. The national press write about London - not Newcastle or Rotherham, unless it is something really silly or something that worries them personally. Journalists have stopped realizing that what they term 'stories', are not as unique as the subjects. Magazines are not real life. For example when an opinion poll predicts that two thousand people want Gordon Brown to be the next Prime Minister, the broadcasters assume that is what we really want, and that's in black and white. However, it pays to understand that those petitioned may change their minds if a hypothetical Gordon puts up income tax and closes two hundred hospitals. With their influence, what would happen if the gutter press decided to publicly lynch poor hypothetical Gordon. How would the opinion poll read next time? With the politicians based in London and the press shadowboxing every move, the press believe they have the power to shape the identity of Britain into yes and no camps; they believe this city is the country, but they have much to do before they condition identity. In London there is a pressing need to conform in order to survive. The inner state of consciousness that affords the opportunities people crave sinks more than it swims. It is not a question of soul-searching until one finds the Holy Grail, the answer is simple. I have been with more interesting children than graduates, I have known godlier alcoholics than clergymen, (partly because it was their round.) and I have enjoyed the company of more talented writers than BBC soap opera teams have devised in three decades.

    The potential to make it happen for oneself is present in many, many people, but for the majority it doesn't. Local Councils of London will wheel out the usual excuses of racism, sexism and anything that fits into a Marxist conspiracy theory, but the fault is ultimately with a shortfall of individuality. By this I am not saying that the Great American Dream is available to everyone who lives in the ghetto but it is important for all people to realize their responsibility to themselves and not forget their potential. Sometimes to conform is inevitable. On a black housing estate a young man may conform to the stereotype that society is racist and that he will never work. He may then conform to join a gang and become involved in crime and spend some time behind bars. He may well have had potential. Where did it go wrong? He conformed to the ideology that society is wicked and racist before he had conformed to the inevitability of black street crime. If he had rehearsed his attitude first the fruit may have been different. The answer therefore is not to non-conform but to not conform in the right places. However I accept that there will usually be a price for being of a single mind.

Throughout my life I have been unable to conform intellectually. I was not what you could call a rebel because I didn't conform to a rebel. Sometimes to be a rebel when growing up one had to be a conservative. That was my intellectual rebellion. Therefore as time went by, I lost my accent, I began to study Shakespeare and I sunk the odd glass of real ale. The price was twofold. I lost popularity with stupid people and I gained popularity with the rest. I began to acquire the middle-class label from the stupid people which didn't really fit my modest circumstances, and so I was keen to shed this label more than Judy Finnegan not because I'd suffer from being seen as a capitalist extortionist as Judy thinks she is, but because I always identified with the background of the working man's lifestyle. I was always intellectual however and felt more of a responsibility to the truth than to my background. As my intellect prompted me to speak the language I love properly and try against all the odds to be a little more sophisticated, I paid the price of resentment, not from people who knew me but from people who didn't know me. In fact some institutions are so sworn to equality that French Revolutionaries had less militancy towards their counter-revolutionaries. So, my intellectual rebellion did lead to prejudice but has not cost me truth, which Judy Finnegan might not tell you as she drops her aitches in avoidance of the truth being known about her background. This media philosophy held dear among football commentators and holiday presenters was all started by Alan Davies alias Jonathan Creek a couple of years back when 'e dropped the t on the word 'complicated' in the Nat West adver'. Soon I heard the Classic FM, D.J Jamie Crick drop the 't' on Bey-hoven. It was a good job Beethoven couldn't hear him. I was speechless. Was this Jamie Crick or Jonathan Creek? Answers on a postcard please to Dick van Dyke.

It is impossible to deny however that a person can be judged more upon outward appearance than inner truth and may be considered free of blame if he allows the outside world to affect his inner self. So while I comb back my skinhead crop of blond hair and tighten the buckles on my braces, I will refer again to what seems to be a frisson of resentment welling up inside London's black communities. In inner London there are successful black people and there are those who are not. Those who are successful have jobs, a sense of humour and fair-play and they are fully absorbed into the British way of life. Those who are not successful are so isolated that they have allowed their outward sense of social injustice, however laudable, to affect their inner spirit and so they become segregated into pockets of gangs with their own indecipherable street slangs, and even drug or gun crime. Who is responsible for this segregation? It is not the so-called racist system for in London there are more equal opportunities for blacks than anyone else; it is not racist violence because sadly for every Steven Laurence there are umpteen more unreported black murders in London; and it is certainly not because the lot of a black man is any worse than of a white man. What is happening is that London's black community is allowing the traditional prejudices of the past swallow the truth of a much more equal and fairer present; they are allowing a real identity with hostile history to cloud their own inner judgment of a real, but docile present and they, and no-one else, must let go and take responsibility for this. However if this were a perfect world it would be easy to forgive and forget. A so-called religious value like this falls well on stony ground in the most religious of societies. If the Palestinians refuse to let go, how can we?

However if I untangle my copper braces which may well have truly strangled me, it may be worthwhile to point out that all sorts of appearances leave a strong impression on the inner sanctum in an everyday sense. If we are not black, we may be fat or ugly or disabled and for these we may be judged to be lazy or stupid or depressed. And then we may allow ourselves to become lazy, stupid and depressed even if we are not fat or ugly or disabled in a severe manner. We must allow the world to change with our opinion and not let our opinion be changed by the world.

However in what seems a bold understanding of life, I feel I must drop down naked in front of a steel mirror and pick out all the warts I am sanctimoniously hammering the rest of the world for having. In truth, at 34 I wouldn't claim to be an expert with answers tucked up a magic sleeve; no sensible thirty something would. However I do know something about human frailties and human strengths for in shining the mirror toward me, I reflect an attitude of which a lazy, stupid, ugly and thoroughly displeased person should be. In other words I share the bondage of human frailty and tie myself in the knots of Taurean stubbornness and the reason I know this is because

I may have been like this longer than anyone else.

When I look in my mirror I can literally see a thousand different faces staring back at me, and they all belong to the same person. One day I might scrutinize deliberately for an expression I yearn to find, another day my big, blue eyes may seem like they have protracted into my skull, and so on. As I stand rather blue with cold now in front of my mirror I laugh without dignity at the peculiar shape of my left leg and how the thigh muscle is curved like a banana. With paranoia I look my stomach in the eye like two boxers squaring up; I say to it: "You dare flop out when I have another cup of tea." But it will. I have defeated my own philosophy by allowing it to defeat me. Well, almost.

When I look in the mirror sometimes I am carried back to lessons in 'zimmer sechs' and our Crystal Palace supporting German teacher, a double whammy if ever there was one. This particular individual was like a genial Father Christmas dressed in tight Farah's so I gave him less respect as a person than as a teacher. He was probably somewhere in his mid-forties and in my sheltered naivety I swore that I would never develop an overhanging mid-rift to disguise the fact that my spindly legs could fit into size 28 slacks. For I was 14 and I would die for my appearance and even boasting a waistline four inches more slender than my German master didn't drain my confidence exactly, and I was confident not least because I was top of his class!

The key determinant in physical growth from adolescence to adulthood is the food and drink we consume. As a teenager I was blissfully unaware of this damning lesson and thought I would be sporty for life. My mother prepared very good meals for my younger sister, my father and myself in those days and although I was indecently addicted to junk food, my pennies would only spare me a rare treat at the Catford McDonalds.

My lager drinking days had not yet begun, so my intake was on hold, particular as lager and junk food are usually served in unison. These days it is not uncommon to find junk food served in pubs, so that those that can't stagger to their local kebab house now don't have to. If I go back to the 14 year old staring back at me in my mirror, I will remember that for him a Chinese takeaway was a luxury, but when I trade innocence for the truth of the present I remember that I have a freezer full of the stuff and a dozen double negatives in the brain instructing me to glide past the chicken satay before I fall prey to the sweet and sour selection. And then instead of staring at my belly through a cocked eye it seems to be staring back at me saying, "You shouldn't treat me like this you big ape." This is the price of capitalist responsibility; it is called freedom and it is called choice and it is the Mecca for every human soul. However as every child wishes he had more freedom to choose every adult has more selection because he has more money. When an adult has more money he has the freedom to abdicate his self-responsibility and spend it on Chinese takeaways. With the population over sizing quicker than it takes to down two Big Macs, it is worth reminding oneself that with choice there comes more choice. We must be aware of extremity.

It is tempting in adulthood's formative years to agree to what you think you want rather than what you actually need. In my case I couldn't say no to chocolate and along with no culinary knowledge it proved to be my nemesis. It is true of many new adults that as hormones change so does metabolism. I knew that if you said yes to three Mars bars when you were fourteen, you could burn the energy off in the school playground. I didn't know, however that if you said yes to three Mars bars by the time you were twenty you were too sluggish to do anything about it, except have another three

Mars bars or appear on Strictly Come Dancing. My inexperience was such that when I put on three stones within a month of starting university, I didn't conclude that it could be a poor diet, because save for my mother's excellent home-cooking, my diet had always been poor. Later my experience tells me that but for family mealtimes, the situation could have happened more rapidly than it did. The dawn raids on a petrol station's refrigerated pasties, which I ate cold, were of consummate taste to the undergraduate and usually a result of polishing off the Rice Krispies the previous evening. The pickled salad lingering in a stew of steaming kebab grease under my bed was only available in emergencies, like when the garage was empty.

2

At university apart from bodyweight, there were plenty of ways to freeze the mind instead of attuning it. The University of East Anglia was known to everybody as the UEA which got promoted to the University of Easy Access once we realized how thick everybody was. Although I was in a class of my own, I was not the only one without a decent meal and smelly socks. The only students who did have grey matter were the post-graduates who could escape from the campus pub into the solitude of their own private bar and discuss essays on ethics while posting a band of Geordie sentries at the door to see there was no trouble. Most of the post-graduates were working class and had succeeded through the ranks on ability and they all had survived the undergraduate test better than some with comfortable backgrounds.

UEA was a mass of breezeblocks and had walkways to rival the bends at Silverstone. It was no place for vertigo but great for panoramic views. On a bright day one could see past the Toblerone shaped Norfolk and Suffolk Terrace lodgings, over the open expanse of green playing fields and out onto the Norfolk Broads. I always found it was better to look out from the plethora of walkways rather than down from them. It was like being in a concrete jungle in the middle of the Garden of Gethsemane. It was Milton Keynes with beauty. When Prince Charles came for the University's silver jubilee he spoke very well about British education and young people starting out, but was probably hiding inner apoplexy at the architectural bleakness of UEA. For me it was how I imagined Egypt, with the Toblerones representing the pyramids amid whitewashed Schools of Faculty.

Everything on campus was built at a right angle and under the walkways lay some steps down to a perfectly formed meeting square which had obviously been thought out by a brilliant math's student studying the civilization of ancient Rome. Looking down into the sunken square from above hundreds of hungry students would perch themselves at a random vantage point and pull from their shopping bags the first whiff of fast food to pass their lips that day or a semi-nutritious baguette from the 'something to do with South Africa' tea-bar next to the Steve Biko Room. (Yes it was called that.)

At the base in the right hand corner of the square was the Student Union pub, which after years of literally frenetic debate had retained its name - 'The Pub'-, which summed up the intellectual spirit rife in the murky backwaters of student union policies. The Pub was one of those places that greeted you with the stench of foul beer as soon as you opened the door. I'm not saying the beer was crap in there but the smell of it sucked you in from the quality Norwich air like the back draft of a fire, and then like all rotting ale-houses, you became acquainted with it and in a matter of moments it was curiously forgotten about.

The side of the Pub faced out onto an arcade of shops, built for convenience rather than comfort. The mini supermarket was stocked with individual boxes of cornflakes, which could last well into the night if one's milk didn't make you pass out after yet another day had elapsed on the sell-by-date. There was always Pot Noodle for a gourmet lunch whose new spicy variety was very popular among the connoisseurs dining in Norfolk Terrace and which for some peculiar reason always used to fill me up, probably because they used to hide the roughage in Cornish pasties behind the same set of spices. And indeed on open display by the checkout were the condoms which no-one seemed to buy despite warnings of the AIDS epidemic which the gays ignored as a Thatcherite plot to disenfranchise them.

Next to the general store was the launderette or leper colony where I would faithfully trek to every third month and special occasions. Here I developed that ubiquitous affliction of 'missing left sock' which when full-blown could become the hugely contagious 'no socks at all'. It was a long way from mum's unruly staircase of socks and undies on my bedside chair wanting to be worn to school every morning. This was about how many pairs of white socks you could buy in a term and whether having pale skin, I'd get noticed not wearing any to the local nightclubs. Since in those days all the lads were wearing ankle-high white socks under their turn up Levis, I hardly needed to worry.

There were no bookmakers in the arcade but a bank did just as well out of its hopeless clients. The Student Union not unfairly was always campaigning for better grants and in the end they got loans, which are a lot worse, and now a national disgrace. I can only imagine the chaos of paying back a student loan when all I experienced was the carnage of an overspent grant. The bank queues on campus reminded me of Orwellian proles all silently making their way to another interrogation. You could hear the prayers asking God to let the bank manager provide another fifty quid till the end of term so they could afford an extra topping on their last frozen pizza. The pressure was immense. Soon if they were lucky, they could go begging to mother and father to supplement there overdraft, blaming their recklessness on book prices and transport. As well as debt behaving like a dreadful monkey on one's back, it made you feel dishonest, and this was nothing to the scars inflicted by student loans. Our line of Orwellian proles is perhaps a symbolic line between grants and loans, poverty and wealth, and sanity and insanity, and all in the name of something that should be free: education.

Above the Pub and on top of another walkway overlooking the square was the vast expanse of University House where replies to all the letters written during one's lectures could be collected. In UH lay the dormant Steve Biko room which was a stark reminder from the Student Union that concocting great names for premises was not as important as filling them; there was never anything in the Steve Biko room. It was just the Steve Biko room. Maybe it was a place for monastic contemplation. I never really cared.

Those who did care were of course those who quite magnanimously had stood for political office. There was not a careerist amongst them! Gandhi eat your heart out. Their corridors of power lined the balconies of UH like a sinister Stalinist prison. I never knew what was going on behind all these closed doors, but they knew what I was thinking I am sure. Were they tapping the Watergate Building? Were they relaying secret messages in Morse code to the Kremlin? Or were they designing posters for the next visitation of the Rocky Horror Show? Which one was 'Deep Throat'? I felt that to investigate was to open Pandora's Box. I left well alone the politics to the politicians.

There were several weighty issues of the day at hand anyway, like would Scott marry Charlene and whether she would altogether take to him going to work on a skateboard. The story was on a knife-edge and every lunchtime at one o'clock the contents of campus stormed into UH and huddled together on the linoleum floor to watch the gripping conclusion of Neighbours on a small screen perched on meccano some twenty feet above their innocent faces. At UEA this was a 'sit in'. Instead of it being called last minute revision, seeing so many students spill over each other to watch an Aussie soap a UEA student would probably sum this particular activity up as 'cramming'. The word on campus was that Neighbours was worth getting out of bed for, and sometimes some did.

It is sad but true that as we swing back across the square past the coffee shop for early-risers, the least populous buildings in university life were the Schools of Faculty where you were actually supposed to learn something, unless you were studying Science. The School of European History and Modern Languages where I was actually supposed to be learning something must have given off a bad smell every time its glass doors swung open for I literally developed a phobia for seminars brought on by falling behind through non-attendance. Entering this Arts Building fostered an inferiority complex so grand that a seminar held all the worth for me as being buried in a communal grave for plague victims. So I hid in the Pub playfully scorning the academics who wasted good drinking time on lectures with fellows who seemed to aspire to the same aversions as me.

The Pub's favourite customer was Herbie whose favourite occupation was drinking. Herbie could have drunk from Land's End to John O'Groats. His intestines smelt like the River Thames and his urine was spoon-resistant. On one glorious occasion after I had passed out in a table of vomit in the Norwich Tandoori, Herbie rounded off the evening by responsibly carrying me back home, finding my room keys, and then relinquished me from his grip, so that I fell face-first onto my mattress; then without fussing he spun round and pissed in my wash-basin. I should have been doing that!

Every year the Student Union ran a year round sport's event called the Grand Prix which attracted teams from the length and breadth of the University. It wasn't taken seriously but it was mad. It was a bit like a team version of the seventies TV show, 'The Superstars', where points were accumulated by each team for several different sports with the outright winner being the team with the most points at the end of the year. In fact it was a bit like a Grand Prix! In the first year Herbie's team was called 'Beer', in the second year it was called 'More Beer' and in the third year it was christened 'Even More Beer'. Although by no means bad athletes, Even More Beer didn't seem to be interested in the cross-country phase of the competition, nor did they show any participation in the gym or the mighty table-tennis tournaments. However they always showed up to the football tournaments and with three or four crates of lager to drink they watched the other games. The team, which was a motley collection of graduate and post-graduate hard men, were also quite good at football and it was quite interesting to see how far they could progress in the competition while under the influence of an ever decreasing stock of tinned lager. One year they did get to the final, which showed remarkable resilience I thought. However, the funniest memory I have from the Grand Prix involved the big prop forward called George playing table tennis. George really was sweetness and light off the rugby field, but his character was betrayed by the fact that he looked like a gangster. He was a half-brother to Mike Tyson but only meaner. So you can picture him playing table tennis. The whole sorry affair started with a doubles match and because of universal equality it was a contest between two girls and two boys. But there was a snag because for George's team, to beat the girls and take the Cup was not enough; they had to beat them within five minutes, so amid the sedate games going on all around them on other tables, all eyes were fixed on George. George was a good all round sportsman and beating the girls was no problem, but fetching the ball when it erred under someone else's table was. This endeavour was not helped by the girls who kept returning his serve to all four corners of the gym. George and his partner retrieved the balls manically and at one point were even crying with laughter. They were still fetching balls when the whistle went for the game to end. With the clumsiness of a prop forward George had left the arena looking like the M25 and they didn't win. The trophy was picked up by the Fragile Balls Table-Tennis Club, who did the clearing up after. George was kept in custody and will appear before the Horseferry Road Magistrates in the morning.

The final piece in the perfect square jigsaw was the Chaplaincy which stared forebodingly back at all the tomfoolery taking place in University House. Instead of having stained-glass windows the adornments were cardboard with the magnified letters of the word C-H-A-P-L-A-I-N-C-Y advertising the need for fresh blood. When the weather was dull the whole quagmire of the campus could look bleak but especially the Chaplaincy I thought which was particularly conspicuous and some would say obtrusive. My friends would argue that I have always been a skeptic at heart, but by the autumn of 1986 my questions were beginning to move mountains. It seemed to me the only way was Up. Instead of being ensnared by vulnerability, I simply wanted an explanation as to why I was so happy. This type of psychology fits as much as a man turning to God out of need or want or desperation. I was shy to air my outspoken political views in such a hostile environment as university and felt surer about the more laid-back forum afforded by a church. I attended a debate voluntarily about abortion in my first week and heard the first and last sensible dialectic I was to hear in the twentieth century. A very mature man in thought but not in beard got up and said that abortion should be determined by 'personhood'. He was an atheist. I said nothing at the time but after weighing up years of thoughts and ideas on such matters, I don't think I could have found a more logical answer than this today.

Fate has often conspired against me and it was no different

when I became friendly with a pretty Christian girl who stole me away from any debating circles into the practice of religion via a mystical union with God. She was an evangelical. Her thinking was incredibly black and white which was if you believe in God you will go to heaven and if you don't you will go to hell. My grandmother always told me if you were a good person you would go to Heaven and if you were a bad person you would go to Hell. After committing herself to religion for life apparently she renounced it on her deathbed. Now what was that all about?

I was taken in by such rubbish and agreed to go to a Bible-study group, but for people living in such black and white extremes, one feels it hardly needed studying. If mobile phones had been invented I'm sure the participants would have had a means to discuss the opportunities to convert somebody and save them from the Hell that lay in store before I arrived, but in any case they all seemed up for my visitation like somebody had reminded them in advance. Spooky.

There was about seven of us in a small single bedroom in Norfolk Terrace and there are no words to describe how out of place I felt. It was almost like I wasn't in the room and everyone knew it. The others were a pot-pourri of intellectuals, couples and Bible-bashers but they all seemed sincere and aware that my discomfort was based on the fact that I knew they had something that I didn't.

They seemed so damned happy. And all the time. The only confession I should have made but didn't in time was that I should have seen straight through this.

I wasn't wet round the ears but I was still impressionable as a youth and my emotions were still able to get the better of me. After half an hour it was too much; my awkwardness turned to waterworks and I had to be led from the fray. Kindly, as we closed the door behind us the pretty girl sat on the staircase and asked me to pray. At this moment I really didn't want to go to hell and I prayed feverishly for ten minutes. Nothing happened immediately, but then I did entertain the subtle possibility that I had met God and that He existed. I stopped crying and Karen whispered to me. "He's there isn't He." I nodded. You see how dangerous evangelism can be!

In a matter of days I was clinically waving my Bible at the unenlightened. It was a complete change of form. I had wanted to join the rip-snorting English Civil War Society to adventure into mock battles and feel a part of our history. It would have cost me merely thirty quid for a whole year of bringing historical studies to life. At university you could do this. All that was needed was a membership of thirty and any idea would receive Student Union funding and you were away trampolining or rock-climbing or going on three-legged pub crawls with the Drunken Shits Society. I was spared such indecencies by deferring to the Christian Union where as part of my beliefs I had to renounce any fun afforded by three-legged pub crawls, although the indoctrination still didn't stop me.

Life in the University Chaplaincy was divided into two. There were the Catholics who crammed into Father Michael's tiny office in voluntary exile and the ecumenicals who were liberated with freedom to speak about one subject only: The Guy in the Sandals. One may assume with insight that Protestants and Catholics do not have a common theology which is why they argue so often, but there we were in the same church with the same god at the same given hour, male and female. That's my argument. However the Catholics never came out into the spacious sitting area and the ecumenicals never knocked on Father Michael's door with a cup of tea. All very sad and not very Christian. But perhaps worst of all, typically MCC English.

The hardest ethic of an evangelical Christian was to believe literally what it said in the Bible. Therefore, Adam's vegetarianism was criminal, Donkeys could do the Rubik's cube, and God loved despite out-dooming Michael Fish in wet weather predictions. The only way to avoid His loving wrath was to be literally perfect despite being a hideous creation of lust, ambition and mortality. My days as an intellectual were foreshortened by the black shadow of blind faith, my reason brutalized by child-like acquiescence. In the pop world, Neil Tennant's song 'It's A Sin' was number one at Christmas in 1987 and it was about his Catholic upbringing. The lyrics read: "Everything I've ever done, every place I've ever been, everywhere I'm coming from, everywhere I'm going to, it's a sin.'

Sin is far from being exclusively a Catholic teaching; it is taught from Rome to Katmandu, from St Peter's to the UEA Chaplaincy, and its one philosophy is that we are all bad like the Pet Shop Boys.

Doubt is a sin even though the human mind is naturally doubtful. If a young child was playing alone in the park and a total stranger offered him a lift home, it may be considered sinful to doubt the stranger's intentions. However it would be a greater sin to accept them surely? This crude example shows that doubt does not impede common sense and in principle, cannot be a sin. But the Church has not caught on. Instead on a Sunday, man is taught to say grace before a meal, and not drink alcohol or smoke and not swear and for the rest of the week he bleakly obliges when in his heart he philosophizes about pleasure. The preacher is surely a shepherd who intimidates rather than minds his flock. My father joined the Mormon sect and lasted three weeks; he chose life instead and for his sins went on to be a healthy 66 year old completely wise to the ways of the world.

In Norwich there were as many churches as there were

pubs as there were days in the year. The churches were of every denomination and it was important to me as reading the right Bible, that I chose the right church. In the end I stuck to a number of evangelical churches because they were less formal. They were also no place for the Archbishop of Canterbury.

The Church I remember most vividly was Mount Sermon and my head is still whizzing round when I think about it. Sermon was an orthodox looking church built in a rustic red brick with Norman archways and a high bell-tower, overlooking the spot where I parked my bicycle, with the contempt of Old Father Time. One step beyond the oak paneled, sturdy doors though and you were in the Sistine Chapel. The artistry inside was remarkable. The man from B&Q was nowhere to be seen. The wall paintings were like European art from the fourteenth century with depictions of Biblical myths and legends glowing like they had just been freshly painted. The whole place was visually stunning. This was an environment as meticulously cared for as any Muslim mosque and there it was locked away in a Norwich backstreet, not half-a-mile from the university.

With such obsessive upkeep the congregation were never going to be anything less than fanatical and here again I observed the enormously black and white extremes of religion. The preachers were charismatic which basically stood for when they said "Wonderful Jesus" they barked it about hundred times like a stuttering gramophone. They were also full of fire and brimstone, which scared me into being intrigued. For example, at one meeting the preacher declared war on those who would face the hounds of hell if they didn't give their whole life away to Jesus. He could "feel it in his bones" and it was very convincing. After the show when he had calmed down and had a glass of water I chatted to him and related the story of my conversion. Out of his pulpit he was considerate enough to make me believe he might have himself painted the Mount Sermon ceiling himself. And yet half an hour previously he was behaving like the jailer of hell.

There were other remarkable goings-on I witnessed at Mount Summons and some of them pleasant enough to be inexplicable. One famous evening it was free for anyone to step up to the mike and say what's on your mind. There were the obvious stories of how God had found them a parking space at work and how everything from traffic cones to cod liver oil were God's gifts, when a woman in her middle fifties got up and sang blissfully to an awed congregation.

Who she was I'll never know probably because she was plain, but she could sing with the beauty of a Mozart piano concerto. Her pitch was clearer and her range more sure than an arpeggio. It was clear to me that I was hearing the voice of God. The other scene where I witnessed beauty was when I saw a young lady sitting in a pew at the front of the church who could have stopped a war with her looks. For the five minutes I was rooted to my heels I gazed at a dream that was almost unreal. To touch her white face would feel even more inhibiting than handling the most delicate porcelain plate in the world; her complexion was as spotless as a sheet of paper and when she smiled her eyes twinkled like stars. She was how I imagined Thomas Hardy's heroine Tess Durbeyfield to be, yet more tender and divine beyond words. I didn't have to approach her for it was enough for her to be there just like the unreal heroine of my dream – she probably could hear me swallow. I can still conjure her beauty up in my mind some fifteen years later to remind me that some things are not of this world.

However for most of us we have to slip back into the world of reality, and this was no different when a prophet from the back of the church woke me from my dream. It was the other

God, the one of extremes, the one with the shrieking voice whose intent poisoned you with fear. I looked round bravely to see this man yelling some half-baked truth that had more huff and puff than Fred Dibnah. Instantly I concluded that I better avoid his grim eye or that he was mad. This was the reality of Mount Summons; you could be looking at a Vermeer then somebody would smear it with graffiti.

Most people in evangelical churches believe they have the Gift of Tongues, which is imparted to the disciples in the Book of Acts. For a time I was no different or wiser to what this actually spelt. Now I believe that the gift of tongues implies a mastery of one's own or several other languages. It does not mean that if you babble away in an incomprehensible manner that you are gifted. However in the Church if you do this, it is assumed that the language you are speaking is either so foreign that no-one can understand it anyway or that it is even so heavenly that only God can understand it. It is of no use of course and therefore not a gift. What it actually is worries me. Delusions do. And anyway, why would a huge church congregation all receive the same gift?

3

Despite my attempts to live up to my contemporaries by praying in gobbledygook, it came to my attention, ironically from a Christian tongue, that I did indeed possess a gift and, down the years several of my non-Christian friends have confirmed this. One unspectacular morning I was snuffling urgently through a box of tissues after catching the university cold when, in the cafeteria, (which I have forgotten to mention rested on a walkway overlooking the Chaplaincy like a pulpit.) a good-hearted Christian girl passed by and seated herself at my abandoned table. As we talked passively about existence she stopped and looked me in the eye and nodded intuitively as if in agreement with her best friend. She remarked casually: "You know, you have the gift of Encouragement." The Christian faith allows its proponents to talk to God which is sound enough but without wanting to challenge two thousand years of tradition, I do believe that to expect an answer back is milking it for all its worth. If believers think they can have an everyday conversation with God then Christianity is a form of psychosis. God ignores prayer directly – we who have tried know that – and if He declines to intercede on behalf of a man whose time has come, it is ludicrously unthinkable that He would prefer to intervene in the squalor of the UEA canteen. However I'll lay my house on the chance that the girl used her perception that morning to channel spirituality through her mind. Her answer wasn't at all psychotic.

However the only one who was not encouraged was me. Was this all I had to offer? I was sure to be less highly regarded than a fellow malcontent who could speak in Tongues. Nobody needed encouragement at university; particularly not

Herbie. I was at university to graduate and please Mrs Thatcher by becoming wealthier than my competitors. I wasn't going to encourage anybody who stumbled by the wayside. It's laughable now that I was oblivious to my own nature because that is precisely what I did.

To achieve yuppie status in Thatcher's Britain one had to be educated and I pictured throwing myself into my studies enthusiastically to conceal past mistakes made at the exam table. I knew that I had it in me to perform competitively with the academics and I was determined not to rely on my wits and become lackluster. A natural wit can often dig one out of spectacular holes, but they cannot be refilled if a little work shy. My interview technique could not have personified the rapscallion ethic any further when one year ago while under surveillance, I had stated that I had not read any history books and was more rounded as a person for not studying. It was the truth. On the morning train up from Liverpool Street instead of burying my head in the Financial Times like the more rounded assortment of egg-heads who were assured very easy access anyway, I bought a rolled-up copy of the Sun for my interview where I bemused the professor into giving me directions to Carrow Road, home to Norwich City Football Club. I figured that it would be unconvincing for an eighteen year old to read the Financial Times and that was the truth likewise. When the interview was concluded in about five minutes and the professor had turned green and realized we had nothing in common, I turned my attentions to the real object of being in Norwich that Spring afternoon. I had come to see a band whether there was an interview or not and everything I did was for the love of seeing them perform. Norwich was just one more city I had toured in my addiction. After forming the obligatory one-man queue for advanced tickets and booking a room in one of the many B&Bs on the Earlham Road, I retraced my steps to the city centre for research purposes. The journey from university to town was over a mile but flat enough to be hobbled to by bike in comfort. The first monument to be recorded was the towering Catholic Cathedral and it was worthy of the name. When lit up at night the view was magisterial despite looking down inconsequentially at an embarrassingly indistinctive twentieth century roundabout. When I had crossed the bridge over that construction I was greeted by little pedestrian lanes with shops that jutted out like their medieval counterparts. I was charmed particularly as London's back alleys were so formidable. This was a new world city and it was more delightful when the glare of Norwich street market opened out to meet my gaze. I could see that only a slope defined any real distinction in geometry between the University Square and Norwich market square. Looking down from aloft, the canopies slithered in red and white undulations like a ferocious sea-wave. And all those underneath were protected from drowning like they were under a colourful umbrella. I briefly skipped through its forest of pie'n'chip stalls and down market fashion if you'll excuse the pun, until I met the fine gentleman who was to be my guru for the next three years: Barney. His specialty were baked potatoes served in a carton smothered in homemade chili or curry that had bubbled for hours in steaming pots on his tiny stove. It was almost miraculous that the only words he ever spoke were "one-twenty-five please" because his meals were so worth talking about, but for three years I never grabbed the chance to compliment him. Barney just went on baking potatoes like a forgotten hero who brought real warmth to a freezing soul caught in the middle of another essay. At the base of the market across St Stephen's was the bank of Gentleman's Walk. It was chalk white and about four storeys high. It didn't object at all to arranging overdrafts for students with credit-card debts and there was never a ceiling to the sky-high and there was never a ceiling to the sky-high facilities a student was racking up on his overdraft. It was all very gentlemanly and Raffles might have been inclined to agree.

Despite still awaiting my A Level grades with some uncertainty, my bags were as good as packed. Regretfully I didn't possess enough local knowledge to see more before the land curved around to the number twenty-seven bus stop opposite a mildly packed Sainsbury's. If I could, I would have swooped on Tombland which was a student haven and nightspot. I have always supposed that its name derived from the plague, which infested Norwich severely in the fourteenth century, but Looland quite accurately described a night on the town with the lads.

For starters there was the English pizza parlour whose menu defeated all but the most covetous and all four bellies of Daisy the Cow. A three-course extravaganza would cost less than five pounds but because you couldn't walk, a taxi fare home meant you could have gone to Pizzaworld. The local celebrity was the 'Concrete Mixer' (Denzil Dixon for short) who could eat anything. Rumour has it that he was challenged to eat three pizzas and get one free in a promotion that usually never got past the second pizza. He cemented a himself a place in history with a temperature of 103!

After your slap up banquet, the student might next cross the cobbled street to the Louis, a pub devoid of what I would call a party atmosphere. There was no character to this pub and you couldn't speak of the beer because it tasted as fizzy as the lager. I tried to stop by this pub as infrequently as I was able, but the lure of four local nightclubs softened my resolve into sticking my head round the door occasionally, before getting sucked in and completely tanked-up.

The Louis was a halfway house of horror between the hours of 10 and 11 pm on Monday nights for about this time everybody's schedule was geared towards Ritzy's student night just one door away and still proving out of reach for the more intoxicated. There was no dress code which made it the best nightclub on the planet for those without stockpiles of socks, and the lager-fizz was a pound a pint. I wouldn't say I was Gene Kelly, I wouldn't say I was Henry Kelly, but gradually I learnt my way around the edge of a dance floor to not be embarrassing. When House Music came on the scene in '88 there was a pulsating new rhythm to be mastered by pulling one's knees up to one's chest like one was hurdling a high bar. I saw Ant and Dec do this once.

To round off seven pints and four pizzas for the evening, one could either watch the taxis speeding by all filled with women clientele, or you could drift past the stone bridge that coiled over the river Wensum and on to the kebab house that was flooding the night air with smells rarely even seen by lavatory inspectors. It was as much Swampland as Tombland.

The pressing evening engagement was symptomatic of an organic love affair between rock and roll. Terraplane hailed from my backyard and I empathized with their blend of melodic power rock anthems to their moving, but never sentimental, real-life break-up ballads with some enthusiasm. In fact it gripped me like a dose of yellow fever. It was rather like Chernobyl. The band had been signed to the Epic label in late 1984, but to everybody's surprise in the business, had failed to crack the UK singles chart with their first couple of releases. This was sheer hell for me as I had been in the Virgin Megastore that very day buying all their music and putting it to the front of the pile indicated under 'Miscellaneous 'T'! But the shamelessly fickle metal fraternity preferred long-winded guitar solos on double-necked axes, to the unconventional punch of a heartfelt chorus line by Terraplane. It was also because the producer gambled with a new-fangled technology on their first album and lost the essence of what I had heard up and down the land for twelve incredible months. Disappointed but undeterred, I taped their sessions for Radio One's guest slots, and talked evangelically to my unconverted classmates like I was spreading an unfamiliar gospel. It got to the point where I risked arrest by holding a twelve inch single aloft through Lewisham Bus Depot. It was all to no avail. Terraplane were not playing in all-seater stadia and so many were educated only by a commercially sounding record which bore no hallmarks of a stage show that made Queen look like James and Bobby Purify. It was such a shame and so unjust, but they did bounce back.

By October 1986 I too bounced back by drowning this unrequited sorrow in a hired pint glass at the Norwich Beer Festival. Now a fully-fledged undergraduate after leaving a genial impression behind at my interview, I was free to sample the real stuff and get bloody rat-arsed in the process! The novices in the student clusters darted straight at the heaviest ales they could lay their greedy hands upon and were singing rugby choruses in next to no time. Being mature enough to know how to pour a bottle of Newcastle Brown Ale into a pint glass without spilling a drop, I confounded the mould by behaving like a city gent ducking in between the medium strength barrels of ales with a half-pint glass only to prolong the agony of a rugby chorus by about five minutes. If I was a pretentious hypocrite at least I was a discerning, pretentious hypocrite! When Terry left me to walk a sex-bomb from Manchester to her chambers, I popped outside to dribble down the phone to my latest partner in crime of whom people were expecting great things for. Some had an inclination from the start, for example that we should be introduced, and it fell to the boss of the Terraplane Fan Club to which we had been individually subscribing to set up a date. She was a rakish bru-

brunette, elegant and above average height for a girl and had a rambling gait like Patsy out of Absolutely Fabulous, which she was. I couldn't decide on which side to part my wavy curls before they resembled a marigold herbaceous border, so like Terraplane's balding drummer I fleeced the whole lot, leaving a tuft at the front for posterity. The reaction, like my hair, was split. Junie politely said it was distinctive and everybody else sniggered at the early arrival of Jimi Sommerville who was due to sing at the university sometime in the Spring. I must have trusted Junie because my Terraplane demo tapes never went anywhere, particularly not in the post to Wolverhampton and I confided in her like she was a sister through correspondence that was always witty and signed with lots and lots of love. Only my younger sister, Rosie and June knew that I would have sold my house uncomplainingly to see the band perform in America and only a man in love would have divulged his secret hankering to be a Terraplane roadie after he had developed stronger arms and graduated. One of Terraplane's later compositions told of my devotion as we leapt joyously from venue to venue:

"The situation never causes me pain,

The communication that we have is on another plane."

It was a love that was hard to beat because I felt no jealousy. My unselfish love wanted the best for her even if it meant she was in another man's arms. The only incoherency in our dialogue was when I phoned her as confused as diplomatic immunity from the Beer Festival outside St Andrew's.

4

Freshers were allocated rooms in either Fifer's Lane, a kind of Ramsey Street stuck in a puddle somewhere in a field and a riotous cesspit of gay abandon, or on campus in Norfolk or Suffolk Terraces whose architect had not grown out of a child-like Lego fetish. I got drawn away from home and got a difficult tie in the basement of Lego land. The easiest way to visit a neighbour on the top floor was to take the scenic route by scaling the exterior of the pyramid like a cat-burglar before dropping in like the Milk Tray man at the screen windows which it is rumoured, held all the brickwork together.

On our floor the new boys paired off into the two guest suites languishing in the dim recesses of where the carpet curled up, and the single rooms were inhabited by a larksome brigade of friendly and welcoming male third years, who were trading laborious 2:1s for uncomplicated 2:2s. This gave them time to initiate the new boys who plugged their ears for an afternoon of all systems-go Meat Loaf. I was never sure if it was Dave's suggestion, the man with a swift haircut and suede slippers because, although most corridor antics emenated from his brain, it could have been anyone making word associations with what had been lurking in our communal kitchen from previous years. If the cooking was diabolical, then washing up was extinct. The problem was that if you did manage to unstick some article of delight from your porcelain saucepan, you were left with what to do with it afterwards. You either threw it away or left it with everybody else's audacious attempt to make porridge with water or scrambled omelettes. It was our cheerful cleaner's duty to scrub the pans and utensils but new ones kept piling up before she had the chance to throw the old ones away. She was very popular even after she threw in the towel to concentrate on bed linen. When she said she would have spent more time in our kitchen than on any of the other five floors, we were all terribly sympathetic, but a little anxious as to whether we would have to eventually seal off the kitchen. After much academic head scratching, Dave saw only one solution, so no-one ever cooked in there again, except at Christmas!

The initiation was thought up when it was discovered that every student possessed in the dusty recesses of their record collections, a copy of Meat Loaf's Bat Out Of Hell, a classic rock album. My initial taste of academic humour was to harmonize on miniature tape decks and the latest CD players with the lusty bravura of my 17 year old record player for bass echo, the title track simultaneously to create our own Norfolk Terrace rock amphitheatre! Starting the record at the same moment was our undoing. Despite making miraculous breakthroughs in nuclear physics we couldn't time the bit before the intro when you either put the needle on the record or pushed play on the cassette recorders and CD players. However like true empiricists we researched the process of uniformity for four hours and our conclusions found that cacophony was not only unmusical but devoid of practicality. The only teamwork required at this establishment was if you lined up in the Pub behind Herbie in the UEA version of the boat race!

5

My room mate for year one was a stumpy fellow called Bernie the Carboniser, so called because you didn't leave an unguarded chip-pan anywhere near him. He was next in line to film Conan the Destroyer with Schwarzenegger but was too busy redecorating the kitchen. Bernie's specialty was like scorched earth, a rearguard battle retreat by the Russians to halt the Nazi invasion, by setting fire to all vegetation and crops as they retreated. He was also our floor's contender for Mr.-Hey-Look-It's-Only-A-Sausage.

It was fortunate that in the midst of our academic banality, there was a real humorist in the house. When Ben Elton surfaced on his UK tour, a thousand people packed into the Lower Common Room which adjoined University House out of idle curiosity for the black sparkly suit was still hanging in the wardrobe waiting to be publicly acclaimed. It was news to me that Ben Elton was a stand-up comic but I thought I could stomach yet more endless trivia about mother in laws and maybe witness a public hanging by the militants and see a comedian literally 'die a death'. I was soon to learn from the routine that instead of the posters depicting him like one of Robin Hood's outlaws, he was an astute commentator upon Weetabix and public health hazards. He himself related to student worries like the communal fridge bastard, Mr. Hey-Look-It's Only-A-Sausage. Bernie was clearly a classic symbol of the unfed student for somebody, somewhere had even taken a bite out of Ben's sausage and then protested,"Hey look it's only a sausage!" After one hour of lachrymal laughter, as predicted I trotted back to Norfolk Terrace to find the fridge raided and my sausages eaten. If it wasn't for

Pot Noodle I would have asphyxiated the culprit in sausage skins. Pointing out such anomaly made Ben famous inside three months.

I had three years to grow into what I had come to university for, whatever that was. What else can an eighteen year old's philosophy be? I have never been ambitious for remuneration, but I had an opportunity here to perfect my creative talent into a cost-effective luxury after the three years had elapsed. My only ambition was to achieve an intellectual level that could guarantee my preparations for my tasks and toils ahead. My career designs were less than vague but could not be supported in the here and now until I had fulfilled the groundwork of education first. If this succeeded there was no reason to suppose I couldn't write professionally. Apart from Junie, I enjoyed a list of pen pals through the Terraplane Club most of whom would have endorsed my letters to them as a bright concoction of ideas and witticisms which, considering I was speculating about a transitionary rock band, were interesting and spontaneous. My writing came at an equitable price by making me a popular bighead but there were few complaints from my individual female fan base. It was good to be alive when I wrote and automatically switch on an instantaneous resource, that smothered the grime of day-to-day complexities when otherwise I was communicating in debased, internal languages, which were neither international nor evocative.

Before the dumbing-down effect of Nineties TV sitcoms, comic writing was at a premium with such classics as Spitting Image and Only Fools And Horses and these fitted well within my own compass of talent. It wasn't mere fancy that I could dream of mirroring John Sullivan's efforts before he beat me to the first punch on the next occasion. I even didn't dismiss shredding my nerves on stage – until I saw what went into Ben

Elton's sets.

While I proposed to sit on my arse and wait for graduation to be a successful writer, my plan could fork into the academic grooming ground for cricket, now. I had already the tenuous distinction of playing representative cricket for London Schools for the past two years and doing rather well. The opposition was always well equipped with some leading potential, it was just a shame we weren't. The Marlborough Colts who I batted for in the suburbs of Dulwich would have annihilated them. One reason why I was formidably strong was my schooling which had nothing to do with my formative education, but my addiction to BBC coverage on TV and Radio networks. The seventies were a glorious era of nail biting ashes series', mystery Indian spin bowlers, the West Indian four-man battery, and Geoffrey Boycott. As a youngster I got to see Geoffrey Boycott the most because he stayed in for longest, which was vital for England but about as invigorating as his cricket box. But when he kept getting LBW to Abid Ali, they could have heard me shout, "that was never out", all the way to the Kirkstall Lane End. Although he was a selfish bastard, he was a national treasure.

However, you didn't have to go far to alleviate boredom with the likes of Barry and Viv Richards (no relation), Kallicharran (fifty average), Dennis Lillee and the mighty Ian Botham. However, one individual doesn't make a team but in the case of the West Indies when the selectors had sixteen world-class individuals to choose from, it certainly gave them a lift. The bowling strength was psychologically frightening with Croft, Garner, Holding and Marshall smelling blood and Wayne Daniel and Sylvester Clarke tearing county sides open remorselessly, when relegated from the test arena to sharpen up their line and length.

However, in the final test at the Oval during the drought

of '76 Warwickshire hero Dennis Amiss was unfazed like a Great War Tommy standing in no-man's land with screaming shells flying overhead. I proudly remember his double ton because I was playing chess in a classy West End joint right next to the T.V lounge where I escaped in between moves during the mayhem of Amiss's one-man assault. The last Englishman to take a West Indian attack to the cleaners was 'Lord' Ted Dexter at Lords in 1963 (and he only got 70), so an illustrious board game, international duel was not going to put off a delighted youngster, himself born not a slip catch away from Warwickshire's Edgbaston stadium.

But it possibly should have because he was nearly a very good chess player and the stakes for his five round match would decide selection for an international youth squad. However his careful opponent concentrated far better on small squares than on the twenty one inch one I was watching next door and beat me unmercifully by three and a half points to one and a half and I can have no complaints. However, becoming a chess toughy was nearly destined, but far from being consumed by gambits and pawn sacrifices it was just another game that came as naturally to me as five-a-side football in the local park or golf. Ask my dad.

He sent me on mum's probings to a reputedly tough junior school to desensitize a puny speck from the harshness of the real world. Instead it had the reverse effect as I sensitized some of the classrooms with epic stories of chess triumphs and when teachers caught on to the mathematical properties afforded by its logic they started up unisex mini-leagues, and the school became one of the most respected in the borough.

As a seven year old wimp, I murdered the cream of Britain's striplings in the Evening Standard Prize, winning the under-eight's section by a clear, unbeaten margin, caning several future grandmasters, and walking away with a tidy sum of five pounds, presented by the World Championship defector, Victor Korchnoi. I eventually accepted the captaincy of the London Schools team who were infinitely more talented than their cricketing counterparts, I did qualify for the four man England youth team when I was fourteen, and fought tooth and nail for my country in the prestigious international tournament in Guernsey, twice. At my peak as a sixteen year old I was invited to a Croydon girl's school who could afford the services of former Fifties world champion Vassily Smyslov to play a simultaneous exhibition, against fifteen girls and one boy. The boy came away with the only half-point but has no record of the game, because he wasn't aware of how good proof would look in future years.

Looking back, chess could and maybe should have become my life, but I had no intention of sacrificing the fun I was having off the table for the dogged commitment needed to be successful on the table. Besides if I could only draw with Smyslov and have no answer to the King's Gambit, it meant that my international prospects were doomed. David Norwood, Chris Ward and John Emms went on to be champions; Edward Lee, Neil Carr and myself were probably cheated by their toughest opponent of the lot: pointlessness. All of this plumage arose from a school chess club with four mainstays whose teacher initially turned his back because I was too young to be challenging older lads. When I started demolishing grown ups he later took me aside to apologize for not recognizing my talent until after I had made my first move against him. When he saw my second move, he speechlessly rectified his error by noting I was the best player in the school. For a ten year old I was rated as the second best player in the world.

However, when juggling a multitude of batons, cricket balls would always stick in my grasp the longest, but not in my inner city comprehensive where we were coached by a rowing tutor. This explains the lamentable condition of the professional sphere in this country. Our school for example, had a plethora of willing young players and we got further than the footballers did in the London Cup, only to lose a quarterfinal to the summer holidays. I sincerely hope that this doesn't explain how a number of promising young cricketers feel who have turned their back on the game through lack of support, but I know that it does. In Surrey they have initiated a sensible policy to instruct young cricketers within their own South London backyard, but why hasn't this happened until now, is it too late and do they possess the will to be patient with home-grown, funded talent? If they have the right ideas to these fundamental objections they may have a blueprint to move forward very slowly and eradicate devouring elitism. But I doubt it.

The scene was no different twenty years ago for the aspiring young cricketers who had to immerse themselves in club cricket. At Marlborough Cricket Club there were opportunities to play in four teams, in league cricket or in the more sedate Sunday elevens. For the lads there was the luxurious incentive of colts' fixtures which crop up cyclically in club histories when an older player or parent is generous enough to organize a time-consuming season of mini-bus driving, umpiring and team selection while combining his work with his own cricketing pursuits.

Our legionnaire was a lifelong Chelsea supporter whose temperament matched the volatile club chairman, Ken Bates, but like his redoubtable counterpart, his sole interest was the welfare of his team. However, there was never any time for rockets or pushy parenting towards his number one son and eternally damned spin bowler because basically, we found it difficult to lose. This was good news because choice words could be deflected from our commissar towards the Stamford Bridge outfit's traditional slog against relegation instead. I know this because I attended a number of reversals with Les and our senior spin bowler, Del, and blue was the colour of their diatribe as we tore over the water below Battersea Bridge in Les's beige Ford Sierra. Like my Terraplane addiction I became hooked into football supporting in quick time and was soon loyally standing on open air terraces in hail and thunderstorms hoping to see Joe McLoughlin find the corner of the net instead of the corner flag with one of his searching clearances. It was never to be, but like my ambitious exploits on Addington golf courses, there was always next week. Even after Les's official tongue lashing when I broke his flask on a freezing afternoon as I disembarked from his adroitly parked cream-coloured Ford Sierra, he could always buy another next Saturday. His famous outburst was "once a Blue, always a Blue", or something equally pronounceable. And he was spot on, for football supporting will always guarantee identity, which is why in today's politically correct environment of unjust hatred against white, middle-class, heterosexual males, it is so fashionable. Because football defines allegiances, it does not necessarily follow that there will be cultural dissemination, although this is difficult to argue after the football violence of the seventies and eighties. However in the alien side of West London I was informed with reliability that Chelsea fans sometimes went to Fulham's Craven Cottage when they were away and vice-versa. In 1982, because Fulham were threatening to be promoted, and Chelsea was abysmal, I agonized over the Cottager's narrow near-miss with the habitually flawless Stills family on more than separate occasions. Sometimes Simon Stills would accompany Del and myself to the Bridge and cheer the Blues on to defeat.

It was a flighty, three-way friendship that became well ensconced in beer, women, and football song by its conclusion in 1986. If we overdid the revelry, we all rid ourselves of personal caution for the youthful taste of non-conformity. And if we were a bit too vulgar the night before after squeezing into Del's bedroom for the night, there would always be Les's cursory awakenings with a cooked breakfast and his consternated insistence that, "it smells like a bloody brewery in here!"

One Christmas, Del and Simon had formed a secret pact to get me to agree to transport any item of clothing into Loftus Road for the seasonal fixture against QPR, and my assent was given on the grounds that they would do likewise. Unfortunately they didn't stand out in their brand new Adidas T-shirts and Gabicci woolens, but I did in a pair of Les's old underpants with the slogan 'Merry Xmas Rob, You Bum!' scribbled on the rear, which I paraded outside my Mr Byrite 201's on the London underground and inside the stadium. The police were not interested in such filth.

However, the leotards did come in useful at Marlborough's annual New Year's dinner and dance, a few days later, when the three of us performed Ravel's Bolero by one Jayne Torvill and two Christopher Deans. It was just as well after the cabaret!

While Del and myself were slickly pulping all cricketing opposition, Simon was afforded an honorary Marlborough status being a non-cricketer and frankly, bloody useless. However his legendary handful of starts are still remembered fondly in Boro folklore for those of us lucky enough to have been present. Simon was an anti-Thatcherite rebel communist who adulated Billy Bragg. He thought his bat was an electric guitar and before returning to a hushed pavilion as Ian Botham had at Lords in 1981 with a streaky single, he had actually tried to play his bat with his teeth, and its never a good idea to take guard with your mouth gaping. The only other fond memory of his was when he got asked to play for the opposition because they were short and he took three catches. Les gave him the third degree and substituted him!

In the 1984 cricket season, I was batting like the combined West Indian middle order who were demolishing England by five rubbers to nil. Isaac Vivian Alexander Richards was chief destroyer and a pleasure and inspiration to those exasperated by mind-numbing industry at the batting crease. What Viv Richards transmitted was pure confidence of mind and body, and in that golden summer he affected my personal self-belief like I was his carbon copy. Sometimes I would swagger lazily out to bat, which automatically put the opposition on the back foot, and I would instantly relax to show the bowler I did not fear his armoury. This was Viv's attitude and it worked!

At no other point of that season was Viv's positive mental attitude needed more than in its climax. Marlborough had already pocketed the zany, sloggers leagues and cups, but without the Dulwich Invitation Declaration Cup our trophy cabinet would have been incomplete. It was down to the wire with Beckenham and Marlborough on equal points, so to assure ourselves of overall victory we had to beat Honor Oak who would rather have gone punting on the Titanic than surrender in the final afternoon fixture. Unfortunately in their first innings, this became all too apparent. In all afternoon cricket, the side who bats first is obliged to declare their innings when the captain is happy with the score. However this is purely etiquette based on hundreds of years of moral duty between club cricketers and it is by no means a rule. Therefore it was decided in the Honor Oak dressing room that if they could stay in at the crease, there would be no honourable declaration to their innings until our reply would be forfeit due to time constraints, thereby sharing the spoils and costing us the championship. There was nearly all-out war, particularly after taking five wickets in four hours and with 'Gunner' Gorman doing his Clive Dunn impressions, pretending to shoot mock fuzzy-wuzzies in the clouds, we had almost given in. Our sarcastic applause for a back to the wall, five hour half century for one of their batsmen was a touching moment. We couldn't have been proud. Or touched.

However in a blind moment of conscience, they cracked first and declared leaving a 'gettable' 150 in 10 overs, a total which had taken them 70 overs to reach. Not wanting to incur the wrath of the league committee, their gamble totally backfired. I was like Viv Richards just having received a parking ticket and Gorman was like Clive Lloyd, who had traded his antiquarian, steel-rimmed glasses for Viv's unbelievable eyesight which was powerful enough to recognize a face in the crowd from the middle of the wicket. It was a triumph of fireworks over adversary, and we won after eight overs short of a maiden. Beckenham lost to Spencer anyway and justice was ours.

I stepped up in class that season to play representative cricket for London Schools and my first taste of staring behind me to see the hard ball sting the wicket-keepers gloves before I had played my stroke was against Somerset Young Cricketers, whose undoubted star was a fellow called 'Atkinson'. His career was to be cut short by a back injury, which meant he was only bowling at three-quarter pace, as I 'played and missed' my way to an undashing seventy-five. After feeling quietly pleased in the tea interval with my dogged resolution and been congratulated by my disbelieving team-mates, Atkinson strode from the cricketer's mess after a Mr Kipling's fondant fancy or two to disdainfully smash our bowlers out of the park. His bowling was mere understudy to his batting! It was thus how I realized my own limitations as an unremarkable cricketer.

However with noises being made by our mercurial coach about innings' of flair against Kent, Surrey and Sussex Young Cricketers, by a sixteen-year-old protégé from a common background, I was being happily touted as a future England star. I was familiarized with the county circuit by now, and wasn't deserving of Mr. Gifford's unfound faith particularly after viewing Atkinson's performance, but the statistics didn't prove that I was merely a batsman of application.

The Lords' ground staff were understandably anxious to try out a run-machine who might just be another Brian Lara and invited me to net at their Indoor Cricket School with the big boys, under the only watchful eye of ex-Northamptonshire and England sensation Colin Milburn. Although I was impressed by him as a bloke, the privilege was a little lost on my cocky shoulders that I was being coached by one of the all-time great cricketers whose car accident in the sixties had robbed England of a potential Denis Compton. I never really understood at the time what an honour it was to be sharing the same twenty two yards of green matting with Milburn. But now I cherish it knowing that my parents generation of club cricketers would give anything to be affably taught by him in his considerable flesh.

However I was still to be mortalised by the new breed of hero whose initiation ceremony was to castle my stumps six times by spearing yorkers that whistled under my guard. There were more red marks on my face than on my bat and when it was over, the only connection it made all evening was with the dressing room wall. Although a prerequisite by Marlborough standards, even Carole Smilie would refrain from sand boarding dented, hallowed plasterboard at the Home of Cricket because it is impeachable there by death. When I returned for the remaining few overs, the awe in which I held Milburn was about to shudderingly fade as he set to perfect my bowling action. I felt like a clown being laughed at by children in a circus ring with bowlers there hissing like human cannonballs and batsmen weaving like acrobats to avoid their shot. I could sense all the MCC coaches crossing out my lauded name as just another chancer to be humbled. I even heard that the pop-star, Sting had been grimacing at my fortunes from the viewing balcony upstairs and buzzed off. The two hour stint closed and Milburn called the group together for one final piece of advice and to thank them for their participation. As we turned to pack our stuff, the coach swiveled round casually and asked, "Who's the one I've been hearing about who got all the runs last season?" The eight trialists pointed disrespectfully at me. Milburn's reply restored my tarnished reputation. "Aye", he said in his dry Geordie dialect. "Some people can do it out in the middle." And despite my torrid failure to impress, a notch had been made on my bat for the first time that evening.

I could have crooned about my pedigree as I began my quest for professional recognition at the university trials that Winter but I decided to not leave my calling card immediately. Those who had shone at representative level unveiled their hands early, with a smirk and a wink among the fraternity of officer material whose credentials they were hoping to damn before the outbreak of Spring. Mr. Payton my schooling Svengali, practically gave up walloping me with his own cricket bat to agitate my excellence by selling myself, but I haven't ever been one to use words before I settle my ambitions, only after when I have satisfied the standards I owe to myself. However, as soon as the cricket season arrived by April I was selected to take part for the second eleven as a second string bowler. When the ball is in my hand it always feels like a mobile phone, but fortunately I batted respectably to underline my credentials that nobody knew I had, and I appeased the wagging finger in my head remarking that Mr. Payton had told you so. The second team started better than the first team because they were brimming with ambivalent, unsung heroes whom had all kept their mouths shut about their exploits during the Winter. Herbie, for example would prefer to boast about his beer consumption, than the fact that he could contend with William Tell for accuracy, and Ben Nicholas was too modest to brag that future Channel Four anchorman Mark Nicholas was his elder brother. Our team was eleven nobodies, all allied to the fact that we had nothing to shout about. We progressed to the last sixteen of the Universities' Cup and the name-droppers were soundly thrashed before their records could talk. It proved an embarrassing lesson for those who shone purely in the non-combative indoor school and I felt vindicated to have not spoken up about my obvious merits. However if the entire squad had made their voices heard then perhaps they would have strengthened the top boys and struck a surer equilibrium in the whole club set up. When balance was finally affirmed in the University Cricket Club, the old guard were pushed down to a lower level and did make way for the new breed who were elevated to a higher echelon, but by then both sides had exited the cup and had nothing but local friendly fixtures to engage in for the rest of the season. My application for sporting advancement through the ranks to the professional sphere had been shredded in a wasted year I had to catch up with.

However, I learned a lot in those drifting months from another unassuming hero whose talent was a force to be reckoned with. He was the university Midas boy who was built like Becker and beautiful like Beckham. He had so many distractions to take his mind off cricket it seemed sometimes that he wasn't playing at all, but when he did join in his impact was lethal. If there was a team of Hammersleys against a team of Atkinsons, it would be a case of the Bugs Bunnies toying with the Daffy Ducks and then going off to field at deep fine leg as quiet as Mickey Mouse. Then while shivering in his three club sweaters he could field the ball on the outskirts of the boundary, and return it to the bails seventy yards away with a casual flick of the right wrist and walk with his head bowed back to his original position still with his arms folded looking totally disinterested in the state of the match. He was so extraordinarily gifted you wanted to strike him so that at least you might wake him up but in the end he still wouldn't have complained. As it was I could only laugh about how good he would have been if he had taken the game or anything seriously. When Ian Botham connected with the middle of the bat, the ball would steeple out of sight; I once saw Hammersley edge a ball he was directing over the square leg boundary, clear the off-side boundary by thirty feet. Botham might as well have been the bowler.

However despite my puny resemblance to the big man, my batting application was rewarded as the first player of the year in UEACC history in 1987. Hammersley was genuinely modest because he was probably thinking about a round the world yacht trip if he could squeeze it into his busy rugby, athletics and soccer schedule. I would have felt no less privileged to have been presented with the trophy by him as I did when Victor Korchnoi honoured the chess champion in 1975. However the only blurred memory I have is of some fool in a black and grey chequered corduroy suit, telling the diners that he loved them all in a distinguished speech perhaps fitting for a 'top man'.

Cricket began to take precedence over my studies because I could afford the luxury of undermining honest research with a well-healed understanding of the subject, which just scraped the required grades. However the university afforded plenty of scope to try other activities and this I did in my second year when my flat-mate, Mark, invited me to take up the mat and walk into martial arts. I think he had enough of living with me and wanted to beat me to a pulp, which he did every Tuesday and Thursday between six and eight. It was a formal education to not mess with anybody from Cannock. I enjoyed my training despite this and could hold my own when sparring with the black belts, only to be larruped by Mark who had had enough of living with me. On some occasions when a computer virus may have ruined some intricate research, Mark would chase me around the gym while twenty other fighters were dallying in some non-contact sparring in an inner circle. The tutor who regularly picked on me to give a demonstration would sometimes announce that he would like to see "some light sparring". Then just before it was about to kick off he would glare at Mark and I and say, "and I mean light sparring." And seconds later Mark would be chasing me all around the gym again while the other fighters dallied in their inner circle.

I only ever participated in one competition and in the first round I drew Mark who was still living with me and looking forward to the bout enormously. My game plan was simply to delay the inevitable, not get any teeth dislodged and try and stay within the confines of the arena. After twenty cautionary seconds neither of us had laid a scoring blow and I let fly with a crescent kick which is not usually practiced and easily defended if you've seen it coming. Unfortunately for my opponent the speed of the kick took him by surprise. In fact it couched so sweetly in his chest that it took us both by surprise. We both blinked in disbelief when the point was confirmed. It was the first occasion I had ever laid a finger on him and my immediate reaction was to think that my dues if they hadn't been paid in the preliminaries to this encounter would certainly be paid in the aftermath. Mark was gracious enough in defeat but probably felt like George Foreman who quit boxing when he lost to Muhammed Ali in Zaire. Being from Cannock couldn't have cushioned the blow for they lose about as many scraps as the Romans.

That same year thirty history students were packed off to perfect their peerless application of the French language for a month long sabbatical and return revitalized with a collage of research on which to build a ten-thousand word dissertation. Once ensconced on the third floor of our youth hostel we did in fact invent a prototype of Big Brother. The party was a congregation of sporting bookworms, some people who thought the world was mellow and not orange, another Terraplane fan from Scarborough, a Chelsea nut who hailed from Streatham in South London, a man who had invented a drinking game called Shlubadub, and Seamus Hoare On-His–One-Man-Tour which had sold out.

Channel Four's runaway success, Big Brother brings friends together and neighbours apart. The situation in Alencon was less different in that we shared what we had communally and did what we did as a group, together. Although we studied it and some of us believed in it none of us were aware enough spiritually to realize that we were practicing communism and it was great fun. While no one was equal, we listened to each other, reflected and pondered and then helped one another. It was paradise and I would gladly reunionise with exactly the same crowd to do it again fifteen years henceforward. That's if the French locals invite us back which is unlikely because wherever they found us there were anti-English flare-ups.

The local nightclub flare-up was provoked by the proprietors. After forking out next term's grant to get in, we were all having a great time when at about twelve o'clock, there was a welcome emblazoned in French on the bright lights of the official display. It might just as well have said: 'Get out you English pigs!' Matters were taken into their own hands, particularly the Streatham lad's whose self defence against flying glass led to his swift eviction from the premises and a bloody great hole in the pavement where his sore arse had landed. With nobody left to defend our honour the rest of our group were cordially asked to step outside by the gendarmerie where in the ensuing language barriers we racked our academic brains to tentatively agree that "we are English." Well, it beats Swing Low, Sweet Chariot! One of the smaller girls lost in the melee bravely piped up with "La justice Francoise! La justice Francaise!" It was the only words we could all interpret, so we collectively hammered them with "La justice Francaise!" in the confusion. They had to send us on our way because every attempt to interrogate met with the steely British resolve of "la justice Francaise, la justice Francoise!" We became like a family after such episodes in France but perhaps we were more like big sisters than Big Brothers.

6

While the opportunities prevailed on our travelling French circus to play Shlubadub until well after three and Shay Hoare had finished his one man show of double entendre, an intense rivalry of general knowledge, and not common sense, bred between the Carboniser and Denzil, the Concrete Mixer over Trivial Pursuits or the 'Emlyn and Bill' version of the Question of Sport board game. It was a re-enactment of the Bobby Fischer against Boris Spassky cold-war duel in Reykyavik in 1972, which either of our protagonists could tell you the final score, what Bobby Fischer ate for breakfast before the sixth game and why Spassky should never have allowed his opponent to constantly play the 'poisoned pawn variation' in the Sicilian Defence. Like many I took up the game of chess after this media-hyped event was an after-dinner topic of conversation, but if it came up in Trivial Pursuits I wouldn't have had a clue. Six players were quickly whittled down to the two experts after crashing out with head-spin and their eyes still open looking like UFO's while they slept, as Bernie and Denzil hungrily sought the Science and Nature square that would afford them their last piece of cheese. And then when I as question master, held the winners hand aloft with the lark another little notch was taken out of their scorecards and a mental note made of where it all went wrong, "according to the hotel porter in George Best's suite who asked him this question when he had just bedded Miss World and won thirty-thousand pounds at the roulette wheel." Where did Denz's little anecdotes all go wrong?

However having the capacity to stay awake with these quiz giants, I became educated in getting the answer right to a question I was ignorant of. Soon I too began to memorize how many episodes of Coronation Street did Arthur Lowe appear in and it reaped huge benefits when we got back to England and larcenied the newly invented trivia-machines. With 365 pubs quoted in Norwich, there were approximately thirty or forty trivia machines begging for a cash windfall every time we pub-crawled in the city centre alone. A gang of eight or nine would join in the frivolities, while Denzil and Bernie would guard each wing of the machine to prevent anyone from touching the buttons prematurely before they had thought of the right answers. On a quiet night when we fancied settling down in one pub we could fetch thirty quid from the coffers and pay for the whole evening, but if we intended to make money we could earn over a hundred quid, particularly if you went on to the local nightclub where punters had been too pissed to see the questions appear in the dark on the screen. While we were emptying the buckets the locals were refilling them. It needs no education to play general knowledge games just a very good memory, but the Norwich locals were not quite from Planet Earth. They would greet our group cordially as we waltzed brazenly into their bar, we'd empty their trivia-machine, say goodnight, and they would refill it by the morning. The next night we could eclipse the night before and no one in Norwich be any the wiser. Our easiest cash bonanza happened in Ritzy's nightclub where we extrapolated thirty-six pounds in four minutes answering basic questions like who manages Norwich City and is currently in this club? It was Mike Walker at the time and I could afford to buy him a drink, two centre forwards, a geisha girl, and a referee! Well worth it at a pound a pint.

When I needed spare capital for tasty pasties, I played the machines by myself and withheld my slippery tongue when the team threw up their hands in disappointment to find them empty. However, I was funding my own fortunes without the need to apply to Denz or Bernie for help. I was awarded my quiz team cap in recognition of my services to trivia, by being asked to participate in their four man quiz team which took place on a Tuesday night in the back bar of the Student Union pub. Just to avoid total disgrace the fourth man was Thomas Balls, the manager of the Student Union pub. We received healthy competition and some staring from a post-graduate team, but the results were never in doubt, particularly if one team member knows that Delius was born in Bradford as Bernie did! Nobody else knew who he was, but Bernie.

Most taxpayers of the nineteen eighties would probably like to ask for the outcomes of their investment into state-run education, but lectures were totally useless to me, once I had seen Wally Logan. I saw more of his lectures than his colleagues because they informed, they were coherent, and they were thoughtfully ordered and never dreary. However like the schoolteacher with a speech impediment, the rib tickling was mercilessly inevitable, because Wally had a weird and wonderful mannerism of smiling when he had just said something serious. It was a beautiful smile that one reserves for weddings and flower arrangements, not the Normandy Landings or a heart, triple by-pass. Logan's lunge was directed at soporific students and letter-writers to inject some passion into the lecture theatres, but the only sparkle was the ripple of giggling that enwrapped the auditorium like an ascending bush-fire. It was with some regret that we heard about his former plight, which explained his manic disposition. Apparently he'd lost his thesis on a train and as students we duly empathized and were a lot less hostile.

In the intervening pleasures of study, I took much of my time checking out the action on stage in the Lower Common Room.

In my formative tears my old buddy Andy and his elder brother, Steve had been my major musical influences and if they hadn't introduced me to the Jam, I may still be boogieing to Kool and the Gang. In the eighties lasting friendships were forged on musical tastes and there were many to patronize. At school there were classrooms full of New Romantics wearing saggy green overcoats which were modeled by the French resistance girls in BBC sit-com, 'Allo Allo!'; there were white soul-boys looking effeminate in their pink Lyle and Scott jumpers, and there were the greasy head bangers, usually intellectual and the first voices to break in the class. Andy introduced me to metal shortly after his voice broke and I first saw Terraplane at the Marquee in 1984, not long after I had won my adolescent stripes.

I saw many top-notch rock bands at university, but I will always remember T'Pau who had a massive number one hit called 'China In Your Hand', because I was infatuated by ginger firework, Carol Decker. What she lacked in Barbie Doll features she made up in towering lyrics and meaning that drew her magnetically near to my own grievances which she believed in as intellectually important. T'Pau were a band with a message all dressed up in soft lights and rock pyrotechnics. Decker is a celebrity I've always wished to meet, and I won't be disappointed if she isn't dressed to kill, like when she bumped into my friend, the incumbent Student Union President person, Albie Davies who not recognizing her without make-up, politely asked her who she was when she sauntered into his office. Carol politely corrected him by replying "I'm Carol Decker. Who are you?" Only true stardom could have made Albie feel that small and that's why she was china in my hands.

Despite his voice not breaking until well into his fourteenth year, Andy was already mature enough to start dating before I did. For a couple of years in musical terms he had the beastly gusto of Beethoven and I had the sublimity of Mozart, which consequently made him far more appealing to the opposite sex. He certainly had the fun and I had less danger, which fits our characters, and certainly entails few regrets on either side. While Andy was enjoying the fruits of a post-coital relationship and had a job that no YTS scheme could match, I was fumbling around a few holes in the mixed sixth form bike-sheds. I am prepared to believe that I was something of a catch at this time, but I made no effort to woo with a dedicated appearance. I fancied myself too much to suffer teenage angst frailties. Consequently, my casual clothes were cheap and corny, my blonde hair sometimes just sat like a wild thorn bush, and my zits were the size of Pompeii. However I was in love with myself and every time I looked in the mirror, I laughed off these unwelcome deformities with a hunky smile and an inner knowledge that what lay beneath was alright. I was of model height and width, and beautiful or so I thought, but I also carried a natural wit and out-going confidence, which brought me endearing recognition from adults as well as teenagers.

My first serious relationship was a total carry-on. The girl only began to like me after we'd split up. Her mission from the outset was to date Marcus a cricketing friend who everyone in the club nicknamed 'Gorgeous' because of his unlimited supply of macho cool and sophistication. In messing around with me for a couple of months she got introduced to Marcus and dated him for a long period, without so much as an acknowledgement for the debt she owed me.

Andy and Jean comforted me under their wing in the winter months, before I made another mistimed tackle on her best friend Demi. She had been another face in the Terraplane crowd when our paths last crossed, but while I had been tossed around the venue like a novice ice-skater on thin ice, that face, and body, had been discreetly observed. As Andy's best mate and Jean's best mate when our paths next met, I did the decent thing and bought her a bar of chocolate. It had to be love. For a few weeks my feet never touched the floor, but hers were firmly on the ground. As I floated like a silly cloud happy just to exist in the sky, Demi had ambitions to be the world's first serial mother. Basically, while my eyes were fixed on the present hers were focused on the future, and while I was dreaming that it just doesn't get better, she had a cunning plan to obtain the world she dreamed of. I simply wasn't included in this. However our passion was pretty uncontained and was educationally invaluable as much as it was enjoyable. However, as once our hearts had done, the bricks on the chocolate bar starting melting, and so did her love. She began to want friendship and look elsewhere for love, which was very painful for us both. When I realized this, the on-off saga became as flat as a fruit-gum and I had to admit that it was over for us this time. However, there was always something and we remained close for many years.

Rather than a springboard for incessant happiness my several romantic interpolations had left me with enough egg on my face to make meringue. It was equally grim when my name wasn't splattered all across the back pages of the Times, whose interest in university sports was decimalistic compared to the varsity foes up at Oxbridge. I was in a good scoring vein in the Universities Cup and wove the batting together that year which could all too often melt like soft cheese. Others gained a foothold of confidence batting with me and the gods happily did the rest with some decent draft picks. The whole club took a fun day out in the minibus to Reading for the quarterfinal which we were expected to be trounced in. And after the first three overs of our innings the umpire's finger had been raised three times asserting contemporary philosophy. My innings was approached with scanty fuss, for their random assortment of quick bowlers could not be likened to the primed penetration at the Lords' cricket school, thus enabling me this time, to use my bat. The match was treated like any other, like always, albeit not this time through the eyes of Viv Richards' derring-do, because I knew that one mistake and the match was a goner. After two hours my contribution was a measured 86, scored out of a respectable total of 210, and I had only run out of steam because I had treated myself to Tombland and a 4am game of Trivial Pursuits with Denzil the preceding evening.

Not expecting a show of defiance, Reading gallantly chased the target with depth to play with in their batting, to put the contest on a knife-edge, and soon the thick of the battle became just as enjoyable to play in as to spectate from, with Herbie now very audible after his twenty-seventh can of lager. Our headline maker, Chopper had struck early on with his subtle blend of left arm top-spin and left-arm top spin, but their middle order had counter-punched with a solid fifty stand. It was beautifully balanced with sixty runs needed or five remaining wickets to fall. The turning point occurred from a stumping off one of Chopper's wides, which caught even the umpire daydreaming. The ground braced itself in anticipation for the umpire to dwell upon my scorching appeal and when the lethal index finger was raised to dismiss their dangerous run-scorer, our supporters exhaled and embarked on a five-man pitch invasion, which lasted three minutes without them spilling a drop. It was raining lager. The hullaballoo died down for a nail biting climax in which Chopper cheered on by a drunken mob, mopped up with six wickets for eighty-one runs, to see Reading sportingly fall ten runs shy of their target. Chopper's unmiserly but masterly figures were featured in the Times, so Herbie and Co awarded me as their Man of the

Match, which cost me a round of drinks.

We knew what was coming in the semi-final, as the rewards for a ragged band of amateurs couldn't have been higher. Only winning the Cup could surpass the honour of playing Durham, captained by boy-wonder Nasser Hussain and his county brigadiers, Tim O'Gorman of Derbyshire, James Boiling of Surrey and Martin Spite of Sussex. But all the pre-match discussions excitedly reflected on the current England captain who then was already being touted for an international call-up to the West Indies. The name of Nasser Hussain had been no stranger to the London Schoolboy bowlers who kindly informed me in a whispered hush, that he was the one batsman on the junior scene who could knock my batting for a straight six. Thus the fixture held added interest for me, and we couldn't wait to sink our teeth into a mighty team whose players must be overconfident for their field exercise on Salisbury Plain.

It didn't seem real when John Price, captain of UEACC and Nasser Hussain captain of England tossed up in the middle on a stirring day of cloud-cover and spots of rain but it did actually happen. We were asked to bat first and lost three wickets in the first three overs as we did at Reading. However, unlike at Reading I lost my off stump second ball to an awful shot from an even better delivery which even Hussain applauded, by winking at his Young England colleague. Although we rescued the devastation we were dismissed before lunch for an insubstantial one-hundred and twenty, which had Nasser and his army palpitating with every pork pie they stuffed down in the interval.

I was relieved that I did get to study Nasser Hussain's armoury at close quarters, because in preparation for the sight of Curtley Ambrose's eight foot high bowling arm he did design to tussle with our net bowlers for practice. As I crouched behind his wicket I visualized him clouting maybe his first ball from Scally out of the park for a towering six, or maybe he would just decide to not get out and deflect a few singles around before picking up the champagne for an unbeaten sixty or seventy undemanding runs. Nasser compounded these ponderings delightfully in his first four balls faced. Scally, who was no slouch, pitched them straight and true and Hussain just played four proper cricket shots, elegantly but without ostentation, consecutively driving them to the cover boundary. I had forgotten that even at the highest strata the game of cricket can be that easy when each ball is played on its merits. Hussain didn't have to be Hammersley, he just got on with his job and saw Durham home comfortably, in conjunction with an arrogant display from batting partner, Martin Spite.

THE BAD

7

I wove among the stone pillars ostensibly holding the walkway above Norfolk Terrace aloft with the strength of Sansom, and bobbed the bicycle frames crammed between them on the double yellow lines, back to my sanctuary in B Block, three blocks from my miraculous conversion, that same warm autumn night. The Carboniser had pitched camp for the night when I swiveled the key inside the locked door handle, as he lay in his small sleeper, snoring like a babe in arms. His eyes would still have been shut had I been Lady Godiva, and on the floor by his bed were the remains of someone else's groceries swimming in a small plate of beef gravy. However with my newfound Christianity, I conferred absolution like a resolute priest with pity. Now I had an edifying faith in the absolute, the infinite and in extreme virtue, and come the longest day, I could not let the Carboniser be carbonised in a tub of Pot Noodle for all his faults and my grievances. On the other side of the divide in my bedchamber was a brutish black desk where I could compile research statistics and a grotesque swivel chair which was as mobile as a shopping trolley. Here one could get close-up to the black and white portable TV that the Carboniser had alarmed to Broadcasting House for repeats of Neighbours at the ghastly hour of 8am. Every morning it got more and more unbearable, wincing under the avalanche of Barry Crocker, crocking the hardiest except my roommate who was all ears and eating somebody else's pork pie. When I turned out that late Autumn light, I lay flat on my back preparing for the next avalanche and part of me felt at peace, as if on top of all my great virtues there was room for even more perfect elements in life to overwhelm me. It felt too possible to be real.

It happened all at once, in the space of this one night while I slept and cannot explain how, since I was the entire time unconscious. I don't know how I did not wake to the agonizing Neighbours tune, but to a personal agony of a black dawn in a living death of Hell. I did not know who I was but I surely wished I was somewhere else. There is pain in illness, there is war in society, there are broken hearts smashed like telephone-box glass in lover's lanes, and there are irretrievable bereavements that can seem worse than the passing itself. In short it is possible for some survivors to live in an actual state of hell. But within the two short minutes of waking my bedroom eyes, I feared I had literally adopted all of these, and then been driven and dumped on my head thousands of miles below even that. God knows why He was punishing me for being a bad Christian, a bad person and for feeling utterly bad was my immediate observation. He had to be angry at my unforgiven sins. The turmoil and insanity that had infected my whole being from last night's baptism could not be reversed by any praying and if I blinked away any doubt this would still be happening. These ethereal reasons for my insanity kept the world as sane and rational as I had been for my previous eighteen years, but the razors were still undisturbed by the Carboniser's wash-basin and I used one to shave. I dressed myself straightforwardly and blinked in disbelief but it was still there. The world was still recognizable to me but I wasn't recognizable to myself. Trivial things passed me by immediately. Emotionally I was unmoved by my roommate's 'neighbourly' habits. All, which had swept before me was distressingly mechanical. My frame was bolstered by a chest-wall of unrelinquishable tears, my good looks as ugly as the Picture Of Dorian Gray, like a collapsible tin-can version of Hammersley. My eyes screened a look of all casualties of war and every drug induced hallucination. This was no fantasy and it appeared terminal, and I was only eighteen.

The scale of my fate was beyond the imagination of any torture victim anywhere and I was confident that if they had spent one minute in this sweatbox, they would certainly have ended their resistance. I could be confident that David Blaine would still be encased in this particular icy coffin many years after he had promised the world an illusion. But I couldn't give up. I lived for my Junie, my Terraplane and the theatrical dream. Couldn't God cure me from the gas oven He had turned up to Mark 10? Soon however, my defensive artillery capitulated. My overpowering love for June and for myself seemed to disobey my conscience and be dragged like cigarette smoke into someone else's lungs, making me feel dehumanized and void. My true emotions evaporated with every passing day, leaving behind a landscape of Death where dogs and deities don't meet. Every time I rubbed the magic lamp it just wanted more oil. I was now God's evil joke.

However, to evade His holy retribution, I sweetened the campus Chaplaincy with maniacal devotion, which was a combustion of fearful duty, and a torrid disguise against looking conspicuous anywhere else. Overt happiness was not only encouraged at Church but expected. I didn't want to reveal the true scale of my utter desolation, and I could hide among the congregations maybe hiding their lesser degrees of shame behind smiling ordainment. If anyone looked remotely bemused they would be seized upon without holy instruction, and a muted segregation for being the greater of the two sinners. It was labeled as being 'under condemnation' from a God of love supposedly.

I was also devilishly determined to honour my intellectual devotions to the hilt by surviving the honours degree that I had promised myself even though somebody else would be standing there in cap and gown graduating. It was surreal because I was fighting for the person I was, as the person I became and yet if I was successful, the person before did not constitute the achievement of the person afterwards.

However, I wanted to be the person before because he was my natural self and felt alive naturally. If this nature had changed, had the change in his natural world caused it. Had the open doors of lecture theatres and debating circles ostensibly been the steel bars of the monkey house to which I had been chained? The Carboniser was right however, although he reminded me with the monotony of a dentist's drill that we were in a "free and easy society" that was meant to change you not into a bottom-wiping ape but an elusive butterfly. This could never be intended to be a cage. Self-improvement is a reaction from the right free-will and at the bottomless bottle of Universal Freedom I could find real life. University afforded such chances, even if it did mirror the unbelievability of Australian soap operas. In Neighbours problems got solved as easily as the froth on the milkshakes got removed, and Harold Bishop became a social panacea. For most of our students shared human warmth was enough to avoid the screaming hellhole I had nosedived into for three years. So why me and why here? The others would one day dismiss their soap opera as being as unreal as Baywatch but by then they would be flat footing it around the city lights in a serious scene from a successful play fully appreciating how they got there from A to B. This would be most people's average dose of realism and it makes my unerring slip through the looking glass simply because I uprooted, a little more unlikely.

My knee-jerk reaction for the time and setting in my demise had to be E Block Norfolk Terrace where something had definitely been displaced. I had seen a change there and in one morning everything in the world had changed in me. I reflected automatically that the two incidents must be linked. I had concentrated so hard to find God on that basement stairwell that an indescribable but literal, mental crack ran straight through my interior from head to foot like I had been struck a splitting blow from an iron broadsword. Cracking up meant little more to me than a semantic hyperbole to those who couldn't restrain their tears in public surroundings. I knew now that the phrase had derived somewhere from somebody who had knowledge of a split in one's nature that even Excalibur couldn't redeem.

What this left behind for me was a smashed up person in madness, turmoil and insanity. The switchboard to Heaven hadn't put me through correctly. The freedom of academic indulgence spelled absolute failure to live up to my own high standards and childhood ambitions and a failure to be invited into the most fantastic hospitality suite anywhere and be among the best. I was also a failure to my parents expectations for the first child to arrive at university and I was a failure to my pride. As a creative suicide it was inevitable that an illness of the person would contribute wholeheartedly to the belief that he too was an unmitigated failure. I had a schizophrenia that made life exist on two levels. I could on the one hand be fun around and seen to be relaxing from the pressures, nutty for the city lights and hell raising extremism relying on the trust I had in my academic athleticism, when on the other dangerous hand I was in the terror of a false confidence that wanted to be involved with the discussions on de Toqueville or Lefebvre, but couldn't because my insanity would be revealed immediately to sharp students who would then not believe my other, fictitious life. Thus my two levels were like ramps on a building site that could never cross the esoteric line of lower me and the ethereal line of real me. For this to be undisputed was not convenient as I became deeply frustrated by the stupid me I knew I had become, failing repeatedly to reach the brilliant me I knew I should be. Each time this happened it seemed to whack me with the devastation of a failed marriage. Failure clawed its nails into my spleen scratching out every unwitty word, unfunny remark, every soul-destroying generalization and commonplace insight which I had never even regarded as being possible. My face told the story of this new language of Braille I was communicating in. The pain of the madness was an excruciating cocktail of death to cause fits and convulsions in eternity. It was the very incarnation of God's lake of fire that he swallowed the sinners who had no faith in Him in at the Day Of Judgment. My Bible study referred to my soul being contaminated in this way as a punishment for my guilt while still living here on Earth. It made me feel utterly worthless and guilty because religion taught that I was evil and that spiraling into fornicating and drinking and swearing would just make my standing with Judgment worse. Religion gave me its ubiquitous shame before I had taken a step toward its shame, and I adopted its loud-halo to put the world right by putting myself right with exaggerated acts of charity which overstepped the yardstick of boundless kindness with both pitifully sore feet.

My face never changed back to resemble my love-rival 'gorgeous' Marcus whose good looks some were saying I could soon emulate. Now it looked like a bus had ridden roughshod over it and then been splashed by Beelzebub's puddle. It looked simply how I felt, and I felt like I was suffering the blame for all the crimes committed against nature in the whole history of the universe. My eyes squinted in the Sun Of Fear, although they could not transfer my mechanical emotions in to a single tear. As a young man I had no insecurities about crying and enjoyed it as a release from unkind reversals, and now I couldn't enjoy the release from the agony of communicating like John Rambo, as I needed despairingly to. However it was as fruitless as it was three weeks prior when a confident, clever and talented fresher had got involved happily with the fun and games with his peers in trying to synchronize the spinning of the Bat Out Of Hell L.P.

My human nature lay afloat on the surface of the sea like an unbreakable boat had just been torpedoed, and then for a cloud to yield an atomic bomb from the sky just to make sure of the devastation. This humanity was not short of goodwill or without empathy for its own species, but its loss could not have distinguished me any less from an animal. There were four thousand humans at UEA and amid that pure fraternity was one humble silence where the Light of the World had melted all the candle wax. Spiritual humility preaches to us what we are now may well be what we are later. If in spirit one is intellectual, it usually follows that you are keen to learn and if you are keen to learn, then it follows that you usually work hard. And if you work hard it usually follows that you may get what you want. This is a formula that depends on success. However there is no spiritual formula for failure, which we all suffer from sometime. If you capsize intellectually, it follows that you strive to avail yourself of your mediocrity. When this doesn't happen, you become impatient with yourself and jealous of others who are more or less meritorious than yourself, and then it should climax with you becoming foolishly argumentative, irritable and unpopular. Jesus said that whoever has something would be made invincible and those who have nothing will have even that taken away from them. This is not exactly a remedy for those pushed to the back of the class in the most understandable set of permutations, and certainly nobody is 'evil' when they are the victim.

While searching for such natural truths that I once possessed I became entangled even more deeply, in the shadows of their fading light. I became self-absorbed quite unnaturally and unable to chain myself rationally from the growing weeds of poor observational techniques. Nobody could have been more depressed or resentful about his fall from supposed Grace. I was dying spiritually and waking up to a more desperate person each morning who I hated for being a representation of me. It was this image that was being defined not by the common abundance of humanity, but by a drafty echo of the temper inside. I was in effect living dead at the bottom of the pit of Hell.

The first ten weeks of Hell on Term One saw the most defining destruction. I was ill, mad, schizophrenic, in absolute pain, all washed down with a Bible footnote accusing me of being evil every time I failed to score points in my essays from lack of insight and enthusiasm for the subject that had once been pumped around my veins by an unbroken heart. The subtle irony was that nobody picked up on my lack of subtlety. In my view I was acting immaturely landing pint after pint for the boys I was paying for in the Student Union bar every night and the price was they liked me as I was and for my immaturity. In some ways it helped but in many ways it was sickening not to do better. Normally it would have been my ticket to smugly sit in the corner of the back bar offloading remarks wittily about the drinking capacity of the immature students around me instead of everything acting as a manic exaggeration of that former self I still passionately wanted to be again. I was beginning to grow too large for life both physically and mentally when all I desired was quiet confidence. My opinions in debating circles around the seminar tables and bar tables were over-inflated from the small truths inside them like they were the gunge inside a Pot Noodle before you poured the water on. I developed a raging distaste for somebody as unimportant as Bryan Robson, the English football team captain who was the victim of the Captain Marvel media hype that he had nothing to do with. However I was annoyed that he even played international football and got a soapbox so big that only my mouth could have swallowed it. The rabbits who played football for UEA thought they knew the game like the back of their hand despite their last appearance in a football shirt being as a linesman for some public school first fifteen at rugby, and this irked me almost as much as their drunken orgies I was jealous of. One such individual who obviously enjoyed a wind-up got me so inflamed in the gymnasium's T.V lounge that I almost biffed him. Where was my ability to settle differences diplomatically with an offhanded dryness that could have diffused any potential flashpoints immediately? I lost the argument convincingly in any case when Robson let fly with his left peg and plundered his winning goal from at least twenty-five yards. It was God's vengeance that had let that shot fly into the goal, not Robson's mediocre boot, and I felt tamed by the heartlessness of it.

The break up was a result of failure in my camp and not because the relationship had shown any signs of failing. I jettisoned June because my failing would eventually upset the equilibrium of a mutually loving relationship. For there to be balance Junie would now have to play my part as well as her own, and she would have to put pity first which I did not expect from her. It was doubtful whether she would like this imposter any more than I was able to. Who was he who posted these fractious letters, once so vivid and allegorical and now sealed not with a loving kiss but a cloven foot? Who now padded his Terraplane T-shirts robustly instead of sensitively like Coco the Clown instead of a Prince Charming? It wasn't Rob; It wasn't her Rob and it wasn't my Rob, so he had to go and as so many lovers before he felt he had to leave the unspoiled memory of the old one behind. Better to refrain. Better

I should wait and chew the cow's underbelly and live for the day when I could genuinely look in her dark brown eyes and say a thousand 'I love you's' for every second I suffered for wanting to say them without feeling mendacious at the same time. Instead the high of being in love trickled down the drainpipe of my being before the splodge of sewage pumped itself back up my person from the well deep down below. Instead my memory constantly replayed the feeling of the shared times and tried to contrive a whole summer of passion, now sullenly frozen in a winter of discontent. I hadn't got into the ring before fate had sounded the bell.

At the thumb of the long driveway that fed the whooping traffic into the mouth of the gridlocked car park was the Porter's Lodge, a Checkpoint Charlie for visitors lost in the contra flow. Outside this white bunker was a cluster of public payphones, which the homesick would seek a sympathetic pat on the shoulder from or a rocket up the backside, depending on what your relatives were like. I never rang my parents. I wasn't homesick, I was lovesick. My love however, had literally turned itself into a sickness. One chilly October night I rang Junie trying so hard to hide my condition that I couldn't keep it down. I tried to be as funny as I could but was simply embarrassing. I clenched the receiver to my neck trying to inhale the love I wanted to give her, but I could only conceptualize the arrangement, like she was anyone, as unfamiliar as a streetwalker. Then like a counter-attacking snake, the poison rebounded on its assailant, which wasn't June, just Inadequacy. The communication that was supposedly on another plane became insulting and inflammatory as my insanity beat its fists into my defiled breast. When I accused her of not reading my letters, her modesty was on that other plane. She replied sweetly that "I always read them very intently." I knew this in my heart already because I always read her letters 'very intently' too. It was a statement of love I could no longer make. It was over. Our one minute argument had not ruined the entire relationship, but it convinced me that it was officially off. I couldn't have what I had lost, and I couldn't continue with what I had. My heart was fractured and the longer I resisted letting Junie see my withered and contorted features, the more responsible and guilty I felt for not telling her what was up and why. This asphyxiated the unreleasable tears written across my face like Edgar Allen Poe's address book. The pain actually stymied the willful release of itself. And at Church on Sunday morning, I'd be grinning at the great new life I had in Jesus.

As a Christian I was supposed to be happy, but my happiness took the shape of an iffy clown. I wore Iffy's jovial smile that disguised his honest darkness; I danced and fooled around in his bloated trousers but I was no more than a humiliated puppet crapping himself in his ventriloquist's hands. In the Chaplaincy, smiles were of the essence and passed around like a hat that slightly sagged with an extravagant communion of contradiction and competitive unity. I had boarded this night boat to Cairo too late to see it set sail and was trapped in Iffy the Clown's trouser-suit which obscured the water-tight black over skin underneath. Would Iffy be the only one to perish if I removed his painted smile and false moustache and would God forgive him for letting go of his heavenly destiny? Or was it destiny to let him go?

The worshippers thought not and without guessing that my overtly generous disposition was a suicidal embrace, they surrounded me like cannibals encouraging their meat to sizzle. In a dogmatic world of one-sided conjecture, the natural life of the thought became conditioned. In my preliminary philosophy essays, I started arguing against the 'if' because it no longer existed in an indoctrinated universe. The 'if' existed however more than I did. I lectured my philosophy lecturer after invading his office, about there being a God that no one could discuss philosophically. The lecturer fielded the only answer possible for a man who had fewer answers than Jon Snow by correctly diagnosing that God could only be discussed philosophically, although he missed the killer punch by not noticing that all discussions are philosophical. Then without undue stress, he walked straight out of his unlocked chamber, unrepentant that he had not employed some teenage angst management skills, before eventually awarding me a first for 'writing my name at the top of the page' in a Sunday School essay best forgotten. The sum of our combined knowledge was that I definitely had one answer and he may have had several, but all I could see was that his overall 'several' were deadly sins and mine was the Big One. It meant that his more competent answers would perish with him in Hell like all the unbelieving war-heroes who had more answers than the blades of grass they were buried in, and the civilizations whose philosophers were born too early for Christ to die for them.

However the lecturer did let me into one secret about philosophy when I occasioned to ask him about philosophical books. His answer was as true as his subject could ever be, when among a nest of black whiskers, he lowered his pince-nez and voice beguilingly as if admonishing me for not yet knowing that "all philosophy books have already been written!" It was omniscience itself and yet vacuous, and as perfect an answer in a philosophical encounter to put my God to shame. It was as simple a deduction as Hegel or Kant were confusing to me, and a one-line antidote to my religious extremism. Then without any air of superiority he laid down his pen onto his tea-soaked desk and clutching another bunch of essays, strolled off contentedly leaving me behind again as startled by the word 'if' as one could be.

I had always 'picked things up' and this type of learning was as invaluable as university life-experience could and should have been to me. The creativity, imagination and bright ideas of university society were no longer educational to an academic who couldn't see where he was going. Social contact with the opposite sex was similarly unprofitable. There was no chance of a relationship to inform one's mind either physically or emotionally and even the chances of a pursuit were remote. When I dried up verbally, I lost confidence, which led to a personal complex larger than the self-loathing of any inferior. I could have been George Best and played the game, having a spectacular time with fewer regrets than stories to tell. George had the ball shaped world at his feet and without a penalty spot to shoot from his life and thousands of other lives would have been ordinary. Better to have been there with two blackened eyes as proof of purchase, than to have led no life at all. However, without a woman it was like the bar closing early while on a passionate boozing spree with George. In 1987 anything was preferable to being the Man In The Iron Mask.

Although I wasn't the heroic beer-swilling, five minute essay writer I might have been, I was unaccountably different. I was not a square or withdrawn and after we had all drunk a shady Adnams or two, my psycho-wittering became non-sequential like I was a vibrant bum with all the answers rather than an inconsequential philosopher. My friends ought to have been sympathetic people.

Karen, the pretty and effective evangelist who supposedly bought my soul, introduced me to Mark whom she fancied above me and who appealed more to her moral judgment. She confided that she was vigorously praying for him to become a Christian before I did, which I didn't suppose was to offend with jealousy any more than it made me more determined to seek canonization and win her heart. Mark was a computer programmer and was a living legend in the School of Information Systems (SIS) with even the Orientals eating out of his hand. He wasn't brash however, or a sickly mathematical. He was screamingly normal, dressed casually in jeans and trainers and wore expensive chunky spectacles if he dared to. This disguised a dark horse always on stand-by to run with the pack and steeplechase in a sheepskin nose-band moustache. Despite him being Karen's first pick and the fact that I didn't trust any man who could grow a legitimate moustache at eighteen, Mark became a loyal and trusted friend. Unfortunately just as he was under starter's orders, he soon saw Karen stand quite on her head with love for another student half his stature, and he was last seen selling War Cry magazines at the jilted altar, while her cries were heard loud and clear by her God in heaven.

In truth, although we both managed a real conversion, he and I wanted a laid-back approach to religion, but this was too late because the programming had already begun in his mind-computer as much as in mine. I will never know if he lost some creative flair as I did, because the philosophy lecturer had astutely directed that 'no person can get inside another's head' which was another profound learning curve of technological engineering in my soul. Whatever was going on inside us we never communicated, like we were two close work colleagues commuting together on the 8.50 to Victoria every morning never really knowing the other's strengths or defects properly and never grabbing a coffee together to talk about our day before catching the 4.50 back home.

Gradually I let Terraplane possess Mark's soul like the mysteriously untimely Holy Spirit, and it was agreed to see the band play in virtually our back garden at the University of Essex in Colchester. I was so possessed by madness that I knew the joyous experiences of the past could never be relived by me and somehow also by the band. It just wasn't the same with me or without me. The band although still the greatest live act around had cut another dismally acclaimed second L.P that was discussed at some length by Peter Sissons on Question Time, and now, before it had blossomed, their career was wading among the marshes, with their sole encouragement caught on the barbed wire fencing of mental illness. I usually popped back stage for a 'cup of tea' with Danny, Luke, Gary, Nick and Rudi before and after the show, and promised Mark that he could access all points with my supervision, but tonight I was secretly dreading meeting five luvvly blokes who had become soul-mates in space and time, but not in this condition where like June, I simply felt that I would be letting them down by holding on too tightly. It was humiliating to hide my verbal ineptitude behind several large drinks, which they would hopefully see as drunken, and not actual lunacy. I feared this plan as I feared myself for not having the state of mind to be honest with them, but this was a desperate measure. It was harder to admit this height could not be scaled anymore, than to admit my love affair was over. However, the madness was not going to cure itself by walking away every time I had a crisis. Every second of every day was a crisis whether I chose to stay in bed or if I took on the fair challenge of life. I believed that life was worth cherishing even if I wasn't, and I walked on through the storm with just a polythene sheet.

When the two pilgrims arrived that morning, we agreed to routinely buy the tickets for the evening show from wherever the university booking office was located, and then to leak away from campus to find bed and breakfast accommodation in Colchester, before rejoining the drinking continent to loosen up for the night's entertainment, thereby housing my deception. It ought to have been as smooth as Pink Floyd. After a cylindrical breakfast and a one-hour seminar discussing Judas Iscariot's merits, which could be heard in Bury St Edmonds, we were welcomed to a severe downpour which drenched us before we could hail a taxi-cab to ferry us to our destination, and thus complete phase one. The local driver levied a five-mile fair, which we had foggily predicted to be a five-minute excursion. The University of Essex was so far from Colchester, that we reflected that perhaps we could have alighted the train a couple of stops before, not needing a roadmap to decipher a route back to our lodgings. The rain abated before we scurried off to successfully acquire our tickets from the heavy stack marked 'unsold', and though the storm clouds outside were as bleak as a Lowry summer's day, we gambled to the fresh wind that a couple of hours brisk walking would warm us up, particularly if passed any roadside inns. There were no other routes back into town and there was no beaten track to stagger from and get lost. With a couple more cans of Guinness each, we plotted our course confidently towards the second phase of the journey. After two hundred intrepid yards, the weather turned so showery that we could just about make out the emergency road signals highlighting the slippery road conditions and certainly no other pedestrians. The roadside inns would open later. The dream of one's first glimpse of rainforest was now a gloomy jungle expedition. All the time we swore and drank, and drank and swore, no benevolent bus driver stopped or no torchlight lit up our path to advise us that actually we were going the wrong way. When a signpost informed us that we were just ten miles from Southend-on Sea we finally began to smell a very pungent rat. Using our graduate skills and my knowledge of trivial pursuits, we were reminded that we weren't supposed to be that near the coast. Then in the soggy mistiness, the last-post sounded from two yards away where a saloon confirmed that we were now ten miles from Colchester. With the English sleet lashing down in all directions we availed our garrison of its cheapest whisky, and swallowed hard before climbing Mount Everest again. When we booked a room for the night it was teatime and very, very, incoherent. The plan to hide my psychotic drivel behind a wall of alcoholic gibberish had succeeded supremely in its delivery, but had backfired spectacularly in its method. On our return to the university premises (this time by cab), we were escorted from the Student Union bar when Mark collapsed between two pinball machines spilling several pints of flying glass. Although the afternoon was insane, it wasn't as funny as the British like to equate with. Inside I knew that getting lost and getting hammered was the silly act of a clever individual whose actions were being demoted to the ridiculous. I always enjoyed a half or two in the conviviality of public transport, but this form was unnecessarily necessary; a plan without a plan, not for personal pleasure but for a devilish purpose. At this university of Hell, I wanted to shine the light of who I really should have been on my peers but in vehemently trying to reinvent this popular hero the pitch black cavern simply laughed and denied that he had ever existed. Some newer friends got the Rob they saw, but had everyone else forgotten the man of peace that only I needed to love so much? Was it was my personal battle to regain that radiant smile of beauty or didn't the world need my electric sense of humour and quality of literature? Did nobody care that I knew this man to be perfectly good? It wasn't that the world didn't care because it was never my judge; it was because of God and His jealousy towards the real talents He wouldn't confirm. My beauty was invisible to all except me.

God despised the remedy I was to the human heart, and feared the intellectual pressure I could now press against His clean universe of religious extremes between Good and Evil. All my evidence supported the view that He didn't care when He had boasted about being Love, and that Faith, instead of generously supplying a piece of mind like Scripture dedicated, also ran the price of a psychotic instruction. I was opposing a dreaded Omnipotence and all its Hatred and Retribution forced against the man I knew I was and couldn't seem to be. The new creation of me had more faith in the old one than he would ever have in God and he wasn't going to die by the suicidal hand of this schizophrenic charlatan, so he waited patiently and more patiently and even more patiently for him to reappear. Junie still needed me and she still lived which was all I thought I needed to know to keep me alive. One day when this was all over she might still be there for me. I couldn't give up my hope to see her again in better times. Like all brave trench veterans, I became a psychological casualty of a futile and bloody war, but prevented catastrophe by digging in and grinding it out.

That which I couldn't sustain I didn't dare to. Terraplane's evensong at the University of Essex for example, was my swansong, and through the eyes of objective judgment I was able to discern that the dynamism of their stagecraft no longer matched my gaping hole of modest indifference. They had not lost their bounce but I had lost my soul. I used to replicate Danny's dropkicks in my hotel pyjamas as he let fly from centre stage, but now they seemed to clobber me flush in my unenthusiastic face, knocking my morale down like a sack of spuds into a depression-ridden cocked-hat. Taking Mark backstage to meet the five-piece rockers, summed up the melancholia of my whole student life in that I had to give up something for nothing each time. Despite all the disguised inroads into the wilderness of forbidden pleasure, when the real truth of existence materialized, I was standing on a log surrounded by crocodiles. When, for example, I tentatively strayed into the dressing room backstage, none of the impossible acts of debauchery that day, concealed the insane reality of my expression or my absurdity and Fall from Grace. I had nothing and the sole joke was that I appeared careless. If I couldn't read this hated pretender, then what would my former friends make of him? Mr. Payton, my schoolmaster, quipped that in chess, my opponents (and teachers!) went from "confidence to desolation". Now this humane remark strangled my crippling deformity for all the world to see. There was no golden handshake between old pals as I closed the warm studio door on Terraplane for the last time, cutting a dash down the corridor to the secret exit where no-one could find the ostracized child-molester whose towel guilt had thrown over him, so innocent was he of this crime. I just cut my losses.

I kept fellow graduates abreast of the band's histories from afar as they added them to their record collections, alongside The Smiths, The Cure and Depeche Mode, to give every non-conformist a field day. The question mark after the rock band 'Therapy?' should have been voted onto the Terraplane moniker so often were we asked 'Who are they?" Even after the Essex rain Mark was cheered enough to invite me to his folks in Cannock, so that he could further his Terraplane apprenticeship in a Brummie nightclub. I agreed, inventing the condition that I didn't feel in the mood to go backstage again. It was hard enough to invite Junie, where my ugly face would hound the religious joy I was attempting to make her trust in. If she didn't believe in my failed consciousness, then she wouldn't believe in me. Our euphoric, teenage dreams were already over, and no amount of Junie, drink and rock 'n roll could reinvent my destiny into manhood.

I had taken Junie aside about my conversion to an evangelical, and she had been taken in like the rest of them. She bought my cheerful chumpiness and bought my extreme good nature that was keeping her from the truth, which was not ecstatic but psychotic. Her love still rocketed out in waves just like mine had done, but now all I could offer was the density of an empty shopping bag. It was scary having to turn my back on her like this and depressing in all the tender areas. When I greeted her in the lobby before the last show, the only spontaneity was the tears of combustion painted on my inside out face for the entire world to see. Junie seemed to guess the rest, and maybe decided to leave me there and then. Perhaps Rob had lied about the instant glee afforded in his letters about Christianity? She studied me intently like a used car, unsure if the engine reliability matched that of the sheen on the bodywork; then her face darkened with a flash of pain, resembling my bedraggled constitution for a split-second. She was worried to see me.

I sweated the show out mentally and not very physically for a change because I was distracted by my sincerest dreams collapsing in a heap beneath all the dancing bodies in the audience. What I had on my plate was so nightmarish, that it was an unthinkably laughable illusion. The party world of girls and booze and football had been a real hand of three aces in Al Capone's Chicago gin-joint, until somebody had put a revolver to my head and asked me to leave. Like the unlucky gangster I didn't get to turn over the random card, if only to find whether I actually would have won or lost. Instead my pockets were emptied unfairly and my debts measured on the Gold Standard of New York. I grasped the fading dream of June like a claw grabbing fresh air and after proceedings had wound down, I declined the nonsense of a backstage party to say my goodbyes. When we located each other I told her I loved her, even though this was searing my already broken heart without any emotional content. I had rehearsed this phrase to a girl I used to love wildly and now it meant nothing. However June hugged me feverishly in commitment, and seemed to cling on for the days I thought she would once have been there for. I complied to her honest endeavour by holding her loosely like a benevolent padre. It was over before it begun and I was devastated.

I fitted in to the horror of my world like a devil amongst a tropical storm of angels, except to those back home in South London who stood by me without the need for rational explanation. Andy is always Andy and changes less than God. I can't say it was impossible for him to spot my infirmity, but he tends to look at life more as a game of draughts than a game of chess. He was always in too much of a huff to get checked, so I was able to close the position and forfeit any awkward questions until it was obvious I was playing dominoes. Simon was led by his sincere principles into the professional care ring, where his unconventional methods of treating disabled people like citizens perhaps brought him fewer professional friends. However his growing resources of insight into modes of behaviour made him a benign danger to the person I didn't want him to discover behind the search for truth. For a few months I could avoid the inevitable from being known because he was up to his eyes in a girl he boldly shared lodgings with, but this wouldn't last, so the convenient solution during the vacations was to hang loose with my main buddy Andy, and minimize contact with my other main buddy, Simon.

The horror show had to go on and when the terms finished I actually was faced with the prospect of finding work as a neurotic, acutely depressed, insane and paranoid schizophrenic. Les could not have diagnosed that this likeable and cocky Chelsea ham was out of bread and water, because he had not seen me since the cricket season had ended three months prior in September. However through the grace of his heart that he and Ken Bates are undeniably famous for, he was a habitual saver of indebted souls, many of whom he gave rollickings to on the cricket field, like me. He was the head school keeper of a comprehensive secondary school, which always required a lick of paint and somebody to sweep up so he generously employed me for light duties, which my ailing talent couldn't cope with. I was just about able to hang on. I felt like a caricature of Oscar Wilde who had sailed through life with the late Victorian readership at his feet, only for a wind to get up and drive him back to port. The popularity that eased its way through my bloodstream in previous workplaces had to be fought for and earned with sinister strength, like I was a sufferer of cerebral palsy having to gain respect outside my immediate circles. Such stress gives way to pain, consisting of the failure to build bridges with strangers who would normally like you had they not detected these obvious weaknesses with brutality of words and humour. However, Les's bunch was not threatened by their own weaknesses and we passed inconspicuously like ships in the night. No conclusions were drawn as I kept my head down avoiding scrutiny and thereby locking my secrets under the stairwell in my allotted 'cubby hole'. It was Hell to not exist as a person or personality, but ends justified the means of balancing the books on my grant overspend. It was hardly manual labour, especially when the kids broke up for the holidays. On one occasion, Les's number two delegated that we could muck about on the Thursday and Friday if we grafted for the first three days of the semester. We agreed as a six strong team like we were about to build a bridge over the River Kwai and after breaking our backs with some stiff duties, we were able to relax in the courtyard in Bermuda shorts and Ray bans, listening to the trannie sending out silky Radio Two, when we weren't playing rounders. To an independent observer and maybe to my colleagues it should have been idyllic; perhaps that's why they were all smiling.

My application to the work schedule could not be faulted. With the school opening at seven in the morning, I was out of bed by five, to accomplish a three-mile journey on foot with no bus route operating within a sniff of the school. During the winter breaks I would trudge through the icy sludge along the long and winding pavement conceiving that I was still in bed enduring a nightmare. My suffering was so bad it couldn't have been real enough to be happening, and the only possible reaction was to shrug and be wry towards the almost unbelievable nature of the truth. I had ceased to exist, and despite there being a logical explanation for the Sydenham streets being sleepy at that given hour, I felt awake to the accusing traffic circling the Cobb's Corner roundabout laughing at me like the God who was going to turn them round like a grid of tanks in my direction and smother me. I shrank past the Greyhound pub which stared angrily at Kirk's Camera shop for the hundred and twenty years it had been in business, and climbed Kirkdale Road's golden mile, till my meaty frame met the lofty Crystal Palace roundabout, quite in need of a respirator and a new pair of student-style suede shoes. Glued to the juxtaposed billboards circling the roundabout and corrugated like a bad wall-paper job was a cheap advert for Terraplane's latest which seemed to reinforce psychologically the drop back down to the Sydenham I had left behind, my descent into madness, and the bad plunge the band had made from chart adventure to obscure whipping boys in Smash Hits magazine. My life had stopped. The sudden downhill fall-away of Fountain Drive towards this unspectacular school was new, and my colleagues who sank their tea while commenting dryly on their tabloids which were exchanged repeatedly were no saviours and the superficial drill of my life was decomposing as fast as the Picture Of Dorian Gray, and this was as foreign as Salvador Dali. However, it was all so hideously disconnected from the past that I couldn't accuse myself of being new as the Lord's Bible corrected me to be after a conversion. I was old rather than new, and I was a very twisted and bitter aged man, not a few short months beyond my eighteenth birthday when life had been generally wonderful.

    I took the Almighty One aside about the crookedness of my configuration up the unforgiving steepness of Fountain Drive after work in need of some straight answers. I poked out my forked tongue satanically at His meekness and then safeguarded my advance by telling Him He was mercifully generous to even allow this point of order. Then the storm blew up and I launched a savage outburst of blood, sweat and no tears, which may have buried the Cobbs' Corner end of Sydenham under a considerable landslide of cameras and 35-milimetre film. Even the Son Of God would have got out of the way had He not been presenting Groundforce. What had Ananias's crime actually been to warrant such foul retribution? How could Love send two demons to persecute King Saul for not obeying orders? The injustice was all too obvious so I let God have it. God didn't twitch in his throne and simply fiddled with His beard. He never replied and as much as my learned Christian friends pushed me into conforming with my heart, soul and mind, it just made the crippling tension in my bones more insidious. However relaxing my religious zeal for a moment might surely invite in the prophecies of doom keenly protested by the untrained lay preachers at Mount Sermon. The madness argued that I continue on my glorious path of certain belief and that I would be rewarded in a heavenly flash for all the silver I had stored in the heavenly bank vaults. A fragment of logic advised that if this titanic grip religion had on me didn't give, I would succumb even further to the mental illness, if this were possible. The promptings of God's exact science was knocking down the dominoes of my mathematical shape and my mind was caught in his vice-ridden headlock. I couldn't get out because I feared Him. I hoped He would go away but He was my torturer and enjoying my suffering. The best hope for me was to fight the mental illness as best I could and in that way I could fight Him. It seemed sensible to relax all religious teachings to save my soul. Any notion of Jesus Christ had to go because even more indoctrination would lead to a banquet of religious mania that wouldn't pierce the damn of mental illness.

However, God had other ideas and didn't fancy losing control. He fought back by sparking off my illness from above and not from my inner self where no more turmoil was possible anyway. By doing so my last true instinct of doubt so ready to survive the holocaust of religious terror, was dispersed into a lake of weeping hopelessness, forever entangled in God's opportunistic sadism. The waters of my mind broke in a temporary placement I took in the 'Psychological Medicine' department in Camberwell's King's College hospital of all places. My duties as a filing clerk were competently delivered in the reception boutique and I found the expertise of the three vastly experienced admin officers extremely helpful, and I needed whatever help I could get. With psychiatrists jauntily popping in and out of the office all day, my ghastly appearance should have alerted their textbook antennae, but I was still merely a junior officer on their side of the fence. The rub was not lost on me. It was fairly evident that this pale, bloated, unconfident non-icon whose belly was porking out over the waistband of his Farah's at just 19, was a shambolic replica of the student who had massacred the image of Herrn Boakes in his fifteen year old mind in Zimmer Sechs. That picture of a wailing face on the verge of a complete breakdown cannot be forgotten, whenever I stared back exhaustively at a demand, pleading for his unarmed life to a foreign combat soldier of fortune. My colleagues all had insight into mental illness from spending so many hours dealing with each case that bowled happily through the swing doors and into the reception area. They read the moods of the clients with ease and handled the anxious, excitable or suicidal, impressively. However I was more ill than the combined freight load of those dark corridors leading through the jungles of interrogation, but I seemed to speed through the train station without warning to the passengers on the platform. However I feared exposure rationally, and acted like a gentleman, posturing with assurance. My philosophy was to get in to work, get the job done and leave questions about my mental state floundering if I could, just as I had done in the Dulwich comprehensive.

I took my lunchtimes without company and ate in a mixed cafeteria for doctors, nurses and patients. In one unremarkable hour I posted myself near to an older fellow who was chewing into a sandwich without a word. I looked up at high ceiling of the refectory and suddenly in the stoked fires of Hell, a new realm was presented to me. Above was a visualization of a celestial dome painted like Michelangelo with golden cherubim and seraphim striking the bells like those in St Paul's Cathedral and Mount Sermons in Norwich. The old man to my right was clearly quite infirm and my natural impulses were to touch this stranger and heal him, and before I could hesitate the celestial dome became more golden and more suggestive. However I was paralyzed by schizophrenia prompting my impulses to also believe that if I took no action I would find myself banished to Hell. I surveyed the other man and doubted the unfolding dream of death or glory, with more paralysis. Just one flickering touch and I would be in the freedom of the fountains of Trafalgar Square. But, there would be reporters needing to witness these remarkable miracles and a Messiac healer would spatter the morning headlines before he would be accomplished as a deliverer. That would be Hell, but incurring God's wrath was equally terrifying, so I could only hesitate and do nothing. I just couldn't do anything.

When this charade had preoccupied a somehow clearer, although distracted psyche in the daily arms of a filing clerk, it left me feeling impulsive as if instructions came from above. Faith after all meant deeds, so to obey was more sincere than to believe. Old Father Time agreed that to demand miracles of faith from a total novice was out of reach, so He beckoned me to catch the bus to Lewisham and perform the simple task of preaching from street to streetwise gang. God would commend me as the best preacher in the world if I went ahead. Again I was scared. I knew the streets of Lewisham too well. We had all seen the Saturday happy-clappers unleash some crisp and even melodies to the unenlightened outside the supermarket and still finish with both arms, but would I?

Like the outstretched arm of friendship that shortened up my shirtsleeve in the luncheon interval, I was no more than a 185 bus route away from Camberwell, through East Dulwich, onto Forest Hill and Catford to the Lewisham graveyard for holy prophets, but it boiled down to looking ridiculous. I had little to lose because my repugnant complexion looked ridiculous enough, and I could regain my good looks if only to subscribe to a few minutes of utter nakedness in a disregardful traffic queue. My tongue would be loosened, and I needn't feel depleted with all my Shakespearean language skills as a writer to tap into from the dark recesses of monosyllabic illness. It didn't even matter if passers-by didn't hear me. It was a test of my soul as a martyr. However to be that embarrassing required total bravery that was beyond my mastery, whereas it was still possible to withstand the pressures of sheer, living Hell. I had an appetite for the ridiculous when conventionality yielded, but to be poised on the corner of Lewisham Bus Garage amid the falling rain and bag snatchers would be an utter sham and my adventurous spirit would never stretch to the pointless. I asked myself, for example, where I would go if nothing resulted. As I shivered outside King's College hospital's twin brother, the Maudsley Hospital for psychiatric conditions waiting for my cherry chariot, I conjectured my fear into some sort of orderly jigsaw. I reasoned that I was employing the sin of doubt to put off God's undoubted destiny for His sick pilgrim. I wanted to see my bushed legs jump that elusive stride over the threshold of public transport and request a seventy pence fare. Was Jesus not hailed through the cheering crowds of Jerusalem on a donkey? And doesn't Jerusalem sound like Lewisham? But what I saw in my mind's eye my feet could not follow, and I felt even more guilty and unworthy. The 176 that had delivered me from Sydenham to Camberwell that breakfast time gloomily picked me up like a destitute tramp picking up a prostitute. With head slumped among a bridge of skulls, I replayed facts of what I could and should have done after my conversion in Norfolk Terrace one year ago I could gladly have given it a try, to please the God who pleased my Christian gentlefolk. I had delayed my calling and I wasn't going to get any better until I entertained the ridiculous in His name and shame myself by willfully slamming crown of thorns through my cranium. Rolling past William Booth College opposite Denmark Hill railway station and then past Dulwich Hamlet Stadium which clung to the back of Dog Kennel Hill, I was greeted by an old school chum who I could never fancy because of her weight. However we had always been friendly despite her sly, youthful and sportily reflective glances. She lowered her cards as we surveyed the slippery slope unfolding down below the top deck and she slope unfolding down below the top deck and she whispered that she was alone that evening and in need of company. I debated that she wasn't my type, and not even sex with an overweight school friend would do the trick of releasing the hold Junie had over my madness or me. There could be no likelihood of sustainable relationships in view of these two conditions digesting my esoteria. I didn't fancy being with anyone but the girl I had fallen in love with, and if not her, then nobody would seriously consider going out with a madman.

My vast connection to the spiritually ridiculous grew ever more dominant as its fists smashed its feet and elbows into my crazy cracked up person more than twenty-four hours a day. My strategy had been to avoid religious dogma, but some religious world-shaking had seen that off from the Father of my inconvenience. By nightfall it had deteriorated so determinedly, that I knew or thought I knew, that if I didn't take God's feeding hand I would have blasphemed against my joyride and be struck down in blind revenge by the rising of the Sun. Therefore I tried to stay awake for the longest night, before losing my slender fight to the morning shortfall. In that single bedroom of my parent's semi detached house was the outermost tip of the North Pole. Nothing was listening or breathing in the mini-suburbia that surrounded my one large wooden window, like I was in a tardis of confession. The world was consumed in its ignorant bliss of television, while I stood among the piles of record sleeves and clothing that I had failed to tidy, in a mere twelve foot rectangle. The dimensions were not a prison cell but a Dumasic dungeon. Even my family had been without suspicion before I had brushed past my slurping pet dog on the landing to pinpoint my concentration and understanding for the night on the Saviour. I was just another disappointed graduate, dependant on a disappointing a job, unable to withstand their natural disappointment in me. I couldn't tell them that I was hot under the collar for a disappointing night's sleep. I couldn't reveal God's macabre purpose for me without letting his gushing persecution off like a fire extinguisher. This was His will and if I wasn't sharply awake and keen, He would kill me stone dead. With my eyes screwed tightly, after five hours without even scratching, I heard my parents footsteps one by one divert to their bedroom at the other end of the landing, soon followed by my sister turning her door handle in the slightly more spacious quarters next door. I was on my own and fighting alone for my life, with no June or any lifeline to hold in my bare hand. I was playing chess against world master, Garry Kasparov and fighting bare-knuckle with Mike Tyson. I was shitting my self for my country. Suddenly, at 2am, there was a breakthrough of some light. God ordered that I must walk to Catford some two miles distant and preach the Gospel I had learned at the University Chaplaincy, in a state of total nudity. If I was embarrassed then God reassured me that when I covered half distance and tip-toed past the Two Brewers drinking hole I had been practically famous in, He would clothe me in saintly garments to hide the cold. I believed this but doubt made me scared to try. I concentrated with the utmost strength of mind to perform my duties, but it did not make me more courageous or daring, and the situation any less worthwhile. However with every five-minute ceasefire where I reaffirmed my doubts, I spent another twenty building up the perplexing puzzle to give me the hope to fulfill my contract and avoid death. And so it developed all night long standing bare-breasted in a puddle of sweat entertaining consequences of truth or dare. My perseverance was physically astounding and maybe impossible for some of the world's leading gymnasts, but there it was Superman versus God, until the unbearable weight of sleeplessness stole into my fidgeting eyelids and quite literally crashed me out onto the cage of my unmade bed.

When I woke I was surprised if a little relieved to still be alive, and I felt wasted by the waste of time that had elapsed into nothingness before the next working day. The point of it all had been lost on me, although the idea that I had to shame myself for God to hear my screams had been cosmically reinforced. My indoctrination was now as practical as it was theoretical. Everywhere I went I thought of the dire need to behave incomprehensibly to be brought back into the light of comprehensibility. This is an unequal equation.

Back at the university doghouse with these fifty mile emotional scars under my belt, I still felt able to reason better from the light of these terrible and bizarre experiences. One answer may be that the obsession to obey God principally had diverted me away from the oncoming flow of ready insanity, to a limited perspective of hope. However, life was more like St Swithin's Day than Tiswas Day.

The cricketing career I had carefully charted got washed out in a mad frenzy of daft shot-selection and poorer fitness. Nevertheless I still had enough natural anchorage to dedicate my three-year studies to varsity slap-dash on the open fields at Coney Hall, behind the backdrop of the sensational Sainsbury Centre arts monstrosity. If I had had possession of mind and/or body I believe, I could have graduated to a professional county, but never any higher. This was not an isolated opinion, but shared by friends, colleagues and opponents, except by those curiously in the competitive UEA first eleven who never admitted my batting was the lynch-pin of the team, only alright. I have however, seen worse county pros than the caliber of star rippling through our team. It was no fluke that we twice qualified for the semi-finals of the U.A.U Cup. The only slice of fortune was that twenty talented men gathered under the same roof of an obscure university, that had hitherto been famous for producing the seventies England rugby star, Andy Ripley, and boating on the Norfolk Broads. It may have influenced my selection to the British Universities representative side by being present in a successful team, so I might have homed in on my ambitions better than a raving schizophrenic should normally, but when ballistic missiles in my brain sprouted wings, the sanity of the selectors among my scantily brained, newer, teammates was observed searchingly. I was one step from making the grade as a first class cricketer in the Benson and Hedges Cup but for the places being retained by an unusual quota of professional courtiers and some future England Captains called Michael Atherton and Nasser Hussain rogering the county roster for that particular year. However even in the cesspit of the Combined Universities back up eleven, I was still cast as the misfit among seasoned veterans of bat and ball whose paths had already crossed in pavilions elsewhere.

In the showpiece of my career at the Hove County Ground against a probing but unpenetrative bowling attack that I may well have dispatched for London Schools, I made a duck and kept wicket like a Jack Russell. My split-second judgment of what to hit and how to catch simple chances were overcome by fear of impending death as an indiscreet madman. With the game not halfway old I was getting sarcastic ridicule about my talents from my own team-mates and then when I twice yelled telling, but solo appeals for non-catches, my card was stamped as a loser by both sides united more against me in hate than against each other as two sets of eleven. I was so miserable that it felt like I was a spectator watching some poor, unfortunate making a fool of himself in front of his own crowd. I felt lonely without the well-wishers from UEA to faithfully repay, and I felt I'd let down the UEA Sport's Administration who had backed me like bloodhounds for all my obvious faults. I even felt bad for my UEA cricketing buddies who graciously wanted me to prosper. Such grief made my bat feel like it was as shatterproof as a pine needle. The final insult made me swallow hard and possibly twice. He was a typically arrogant and slightly suave South African whose only shot execution as far as I could assess was the one-day nudge down to third-man. Bearing in mind the technique of my laughably ordinary dismissal, he felt that it required a subtle master class on the art of batting that he alone was qualified to give. This man was no Colin Milburn in stature, but he was the game's finest exponent of the one-day dab-shot, and coached it to me like I was a seven year old being taught by Sir Geoffrey Boycott. However, he was disarming not to charge me for this privilege. In the nets he practiced his perfect bowling armoury against me and because I was more angry than worried, I spanked it rather than dabbed it. As his bowling grew more hostile, so did my own mental fury, and I gave him a lesson of how to play cricket with the middle of your bat, when you are not supposing God is signing your death warrant.

After enduring the two day profanities and jibes postured by my avuncular superiors in British Universities cricket, I turned my back to the familiar luxuries of flat pitches in East Anglia and one or two death traps in Dulwich. Notwithstanding the style, the standard between highly-strung testosterone levels of student cricket and sedate but wily adult cricket was not much. My volume of runs for the Marlborough first eleven was still numerically substantial despite running permanently low on natural assets, and the mind-games Viv Richards had taught me some three seasons previously. However, to my teammates it looked like business as usual, and only I was aware of the colossal creaking's in my old batting foundations. Every sport is mental and the outlook of one's mind usually decides performance standards. It is not simply a question of possessing a game attitude; success can rely on the subtler techniques of judgment and examination of the state of affairs as they stand. I could no longer read the game and I became as disheveled as my schizophrenia afforded. I soon hung my 'could have been a cricketer' dirty boots tag up for the more serious 'wannabe a cricketer but is limited' dirty boots tag, before becoming a jokey 'no hoper', folding my arms on the boundary rope as disinterested as Hatty Hammersley, except wearing three moth-eaten sweaters over five protruding bellies. There was never any money in cricket anyway.

However while still biffing centuries in the Surrey outback my Marlborough friends could not deduce that this writing was on the wall, and these included Andy who knew my game as well as he knew me. When being safely escorted to Roehampton in the back of a camper van, he scrutinized the unecstatic trickle of cold blood streaming down my face, and happily clowned that "I looked like death warmed up". However my world refused to beckon to him, and he passed over it lightly to attack the car-stereo which was more distasteful. If my oldest friend could only wisecrack about my Hell and my family were in the dark too, then nobody had a chance of picking up on my instances of late-night behaviour. This suited me because it bought more time to fool doubters from asking intrusive questions about my health.

As I swung from fooling others at university and holding out for that all heavenly flash of divine salvation, life still went ahead without lending me an olive branch. I had bleakly become the figure of fun that Colin Milburn outwardly enjoyed getting teased for in his playing days. But inwardly I hated it. My eyes still cast back to what I was and what I therefore could have been. It distressed me so severely that the effort to bleed one single tear was as concentrated as a Nazi death-camp. Work-wise it was hopeless, and my professional pride as a writer was dismissively ridiculed with results being assessed as "silly" or "garbled", by lecturers with one-track historical minds, however true that stood.

After the voyage to France where I met a good circle of friends, students were required to collate all their information about the region's historical culture into a forty-page document to be read by the School and be graded for the Final Examinations. All I had researched in France was how to butter the left-over crumbs of a stale baguette smothered in Brie and I couldn't write a ten-thousand word dissertation on that. Mark gave me the freedom of his home computer to type together an assortment of borrowed phrases and terminally-ill dialectics which he could have written better in algebraic. When he glanced around the screen he sublimely accused poor old J.R.R Tolkien of not being able to "string a single sentence together properly". This observation was cutting enough for an undergraduate weaned on the intelligent artistries of Herrn Boakes and Mr. Payton but it went deeper than that because writing was all that I knew and the only lesson being spelt out by it was my own miserable defeat. After being marked down for a third for my industries, there was more egg on my face than cheese, and I began to seriously fear that I could fail in an arts subject which was as impossible as finding future employment. I procrastinated this compelling assertion by spending long hours in the Coney Hall long room drinking pink gins and observing run rates, but in my quieter more reflective moods, I was lacing my cups of coffee with doses of brandy. I stuck to my galactic task, stubbornly to prove a point to myself and the system of education, but I was no longer a naturally attractive wit who could pull the wool over a turgid essay as tight as a roll of string. I was the Garbler slipping below the plimsoll line of freight with each passing hour. If I went home empty-handed after wasting my family's generous support, as I had been liable to do, how would I live with myself? They had more to lose than those in the middle-income bracket whose sons and daughters I knew at UEA. In failing an exam I would fail myself, but for some brief words of enlightened consolation from Ben Elton and Carol Decker. If I failed I would go home and whereon from there? No employer would keep me long enough to interview me, and that included the Inner London Education Authority who Les had audaciously compromised. The debts were mounting linearly which I was encouraging trivia machines to goad halfway, but if I had to support this with social security payments, there would be much second-guessing of why a family's golden boy became a social drop-out. My pride was embarrassed from weighing up these potential future hazards because they left my only positive dimension of hope distantly behind them. I was already unrecognizable to them before these future sins should be slain but they thought unsympathetically that what I had become was really what I was. Once in a restaurant the post meal subject was the merits of my sister as usual, who had been graced with likenesses to past generations over two thousand years ago, when my father stood up and laughed by closing the conversation with, "but God knows where Rob comes from". Then he just stared with marvelous admiration at Rosie. They all began to laugh at the joke but not the truth which was I indeed did not belong to them or anyone anymore. I was so inhuman emotionally that I belonged to the Dark Ages where King Arthur had also been granted an audience of illegitimacy. I felt fostered like a stepson or godson and son in name where indirect terms and conditions also applied. My mother and father's attitude towards me was yet another slap in the face from His Holiness. He was behind her driving ambition to push me into careers that befitted my former talents, while my father inflamed the situation by leaning extravagantly towards my sister who seemed to ignore me. Number fifty-six Queenswood Road became irritable and anti-social which quintupled my persecution complex of paranoia about being the last Mohican of his species. The only connection was with God for all this, which just made me feel more angry with Him for instigating my suffering, so I swatted Him away like a fly every time He called to say He loved me while plotting my downfall. It was like avoiding someone you didn't want to meet on a certain street corner, except when you bluffed an alternative route you met Him on a different street corner. It was a battle of wits from which no one would dare budge.

8

In the final year of my student slog, I came to depend on the friends who had not bought my fake I.D in France as the dreaded finals lurked menacingly in the homerun. Concrete, who now lived next door to my Trivial Pursuits board game threw his colossal ten stones behind my quest for cricketing greatness before it was too late. However I had been roughed up by the UEACC establishment again as all Yorkshire heroes had been wiped out by their committeemen in the seventies. When word spilled out about my non-conformity around the various sporting clubs in the university side-alleys, it didn't make me that popular. A certain amount of whining noises transmitted from the second eleven understandably, but through Denzil's footballing connections my name got spot-lighted in the 'Boycott v Team Spirit Affair'. After saving the match at Reading, I needed time to consider my studies before the finals, which were just two months away. My form was good enough and I didn't want to think too much about it in trivial net sessions, which could bring doubts and batting gremlins into my game. Unfortunately the captain judged that this would affect team morale and sent one of his spies out to uncover just what I was doing partying in fancy restaurants while the other players were practicing. It was much ado about nothing even to my teammates who understood that the Boycott batting school of averages had to be preserved at any cost, and most of them were deflated when I was shown the exit door for the rival clash against Essex. My spin-doctor, Denzil, was a big-hearted man who turned up to cheer on the opposition, while five-hundred other students came from the library to signal their support for the guys, like it was a university boat-race. It was if the captain had invited them there he and my jaded spirits flagged when I considered that I couldn't impress a slice of the university with the one mighty tendency I still possessed after my academic capabilities had let me down. However when the captain was dismissed for a second ball duck Denz and I were grinning like Steinway pianos and clinked the two Newcastle Brown Ales like we had just seen the fall of Mafeking. UEA destroyed Essex with little resistance and after a team meeting the brooding players reformed the status quo by allowing me to join up again for the showpiece against Durham, where I was dismissed second ball. Denz and Herbie had not travelled with the party to the game held on the neutral Derbyshire County Ground and the university library had reopened so on a typically dismal Summer morning, there was only a few cows in remote fields as interested spectators. There was a buzz about standing a real chance against Nasser Hussain's men, but there was a heavy anchor in one of our big gun's minds, sending my thought processes into orbit which was where I could literally smash the ball if God intended it. It was no wonder I made nought, because God wasn't ready to instill belief by performing a miracle. I was as mixed up as I had been down at Hove and was almost relieved to be sent directly back to the warm pavilion. Denz blamed the captain unfairly, but in the next game I made an unbeaten 75, which he yelped at as if Bernie Slaven had netted for Middlesboro.

It wasn't about sport ultimately because he threw me an even weightier lifeline in my academic life. My revision workload was insubstantial. My essays were never accurate or well researched, and I didn't have a clue what I was on about. Denzil had a more powerful brain, which had been virtually on cruise control from the moment he had confidently expected to not flunk the finals. Since the French experience and my horrific penalty miss in the dying seconds against 'Even More Beers' our friendship had cheerily been cemented. He was more carefree about lending a helping hand to a mate than the whole Student Union and shared his well-crafted essays like he shared the booty of trivia machines to those who had not contributed. Having a good head for the facts he had taught me, it was vital to remember the details of what he had written, even if I couldn't process them in my nonsensical head. Then, just as the panic subsided, God conveniently shoved His ugly features straight into mine once more and this time He demanded completed tasks or Hell! The emphasis was again on shame, but the assault was not quite launched at what I feared most. His light was revealed to me one month before the finals were due and He gave me clear orders that I was to burst in on my other next-door neighbour in Waveney Terrace and spread His Gospel by shrieking that he should "give his love and life to the Lord". If I did this I would be restored intellectually enough to perform in the exams, as I wanted. But Waveney Terrace didn't inspire insipid capitulation to my Overseer. The structure of rectangular breezeblocks produced coldness like Tenko which couldn't match the earthy mathematics of the Norfolk Terrace Lego set. There were no pyramids to joyride to the sky in, just a drab looking cellblock with solemn curtains backing out onto the car pool. It reflected my whole fall from grace from meritorious funster to corrupt Bible-Basher, from a young man to an old man. In my room the skulls and crossbones of Iron Maiden posters made it a right old shindig. Del had remarked once that he liked the sinister artwork of their record sleeves, which I had replicated hexagonally on my wall, miserably replacing the effigies of Jesus and a dozen crucifixes, which had shone there in all their futile delight. I had walked in through the out door as a free man but potentially could depart as an Eddie, Iron

Maiden's twelve foot-high evil mascot. It all depended on whether I obeyed God's instructions and graduated.

I suspected that if I didn't follow God's holy orders, I wouldn't necessarily perish as He always predicted. Past experiences reckoned that there would be second chances and I had a good month to determine my fate. I had a slim chance of making the grade if I allowed any distant intellectual spark to catch on the spasmodic fire of historical imagination, without busting in on my neighbour. However, skimming through not so skimpy course manuals while bucking the feminist trend of underlining salient points in gold pen was not my style, and would ruin the books. I wanted to invent interpretative insight to flavour my arguments like the hallowed artifacts of A.J.P.Taylor or Georges Lefebvre or Baron de Toqueville who I had gone to university to dream side-by-side with. However, I couldn't pretend that my newfound strength lay in my retentive memory, which reduced me to, catechized learning, instead of the license to intellectually roam the fields of gold of my celebrated historians. It was bitterly disappointing because a person can learn nothing from boring lists, but a qualification was still the prerequirement.

I could relax somewhat in the psychotic belief that I had until I was under the exam roof to procrastinate. The opening of the hotline did lend me a fraction of insight, which it felt right to obey. I figured that if I sat in the gymnasium sweatbox trusting my own depleted reserves I could fall on my head, but if I stole a couple of tricks from Denzil's notes, it might prove wiser. When I petitioned Denzil for help, he languidly took no offence, maybe even honoured that a fellow undergraduate admired his testing analysis, more than he respected my batting gusto. I trusted his dour pass-rate more than any further reading I could investigate, because the style was simple, precise and detailed, which meant it was easy to formulate in my mind and then copy on to paper. If I resorted to any other method, it would mean I would be the first laughing stock to fail an Arts subject in the establishment's twenty-five year existence.

The sweat began almost immediately with my mind cashing in like a trivia-machine on brand new facts that had been at my leisure to learn for three years instead of three weeks. The boozy nights playing trivial pursuits became like careful games of chess, slumped in front of yet another installment of Quiz Night with Ross King on the quiet T.V that stared back at my primitive bed adjacent cell-block wall behind me. My university life had all come down to these last desperate hours. I had sunk too many pints, set a new trend in vacant footwear, become grossly overweight and bought some quite obviously useless trivia. Instead of filling my noted scalp with important information and gone on to profess knowledge, all I had learnt was quite unenlightening, whereas what I already knew was as dead as a colony of white doves fleeing to a doomed oil-slick in the mid Atlantic.

I had always thrived in a seated examination, and that summer the stress keyed me up to perform well as I suspected. My first-class memory didn't let me down as I regurgitated Denz's factual notes with ease. His marks had always been high and the only insight I could deliver was that I could rely on them more than I could myself. Last minute nerves naturally made me doubt this however. I wrote copiously and answered the selected questions I had set aside my revision for, in each three-hour examination text. It was extremely lucky that I had been there at all for one paper, which began at 9am, because on the green outside the gymnasium hall I fell asleep from the extremity of nocturnal revision. With three years course work crammed into twelve hours assimilation, I produced enough competitive adrenalin to reproduce the goods like I was making a century for England, but without a random wake-up call from somebody it might never have been.

With the results pending, I spent most of the last rites of the university corridor of Time under the covers in Waveney Terrace. The issue of bailing out of the aeroplane and obeying the Innocent One had still to be resolved before I packed my bags, but it was no good and never likely to happen. His final act of Compassion assured me that the room next door would still be available at UEA, even after I had returned to London to begin a life without a career. The neighbour I had never known or seen in Room 11 of A block could still carry hope for centuries, without meaning a toss.

I was still concentrating on God when the result of my three-year willpower was posted onto the Arts Building notice board with the family of others. This was the morning of King Charles the First's execution I vaguely remembered reading about where the murder of the monarch resulted in ten years of uncertainty and I felt I was actually witnessing this death as my own. It was devilishly surreal. I couldn't not pass; I couldn't allow that wall chart to become a list of noble decapitation for the baying hordes. Conveniently Denz broke the news outside the University House walkway overlooking the deep quadrangle snake pit. He had obviously passed without so much as a back spasm, but he knew his degree could never have been in doubt, even after the hours and hours of lack of effort. He had scored a watertight second-class degree laughed off by the majority as a Desmond Tutu, but not by me whose ambitions could stretch no higher. With an unflinching but yet autumnal look in his eye, he casually pressed me on how I had done. We both knew that he had already seen my results. I replied that I dare not spy. Then he said, "I think you should!" I scrambled quicker than Sir Geoff Boycott's batting partners around the less intimidating square than before, virtually leapt over the twenty foot high scaffolding of the Chaplaincy and hastily joined the back end of the backslapping queue for those mentally unimpaired by schizophrenia. Denzil was right. His sincerity was clear from the moment he had called me for the run four seconds ago. There it was. A Desmond Tutu for R.A.Morrison (B.A.hons). I had accomplished my academic dreams in the fanatical screams. I held evidence in my future memory that spoke for every last drop of madness to dislocate my mind from reality, and how I had fought to regain that elusive sense of myself. I had procured survival techniques, maybe even against the heart attack I could foresee from the wall of physical stress that ground me like coffee before I turned thirty. I jostled with the faithful in the busy amphitheatre of celebration excitedly reflecting on my momentous achievement of salvaging one mere dream from several thousand 'dead and gone' ones, and clutching a degree of pride, slipped into the refectory to sit as a man among equals. After rekindling their absolute faith in educational pursuits, my peers, friends and classmates were troughing and coughing back the ease at which they had all passed heartlessly. For me it was too much to ignore the safety of permanent recognition after all the inferiority of coursework grades that had trounced my confident outlook and self-esteem. I grimaced at their worlds and mine, but I still had been deemed to be on level terms with their dry, intercontinental warmth. It felt good for both camps to say that I was always their equal. After all the stress, turmoil and terror, I suspended their snacking knives and forks for a tiny second, by attempting to open the dry floodgates with the vale of tears I had impended. Somebody may have noticed disinterestedly in passing and probably thought I was crazy. To cry with relief at a Desmond Tutu was strangely heretical to them, as it showed up a mediocre non-tryer, obviously at university to waste time and please pushy parents. One of my former teachers called it a "beer-drinker's degree." If only they knew.

Andy had still no more knowledge of his uses as a lifesaver during these crises. Married to his childhood sweetheart as recently as the summer of graduation, I became a cordial mainstay of their first few months together. If there was nothing else then there was their hospitality. With a B.A in History to offer, I was soon failing every interview in sight, yet somehow I managed to reinvent my duties as a temporary filing clerk again to assuage the gentlemanly bank manager from adding insult to frozen pizza debts. I had no girlfriend and no ties, and Andy managed to offset his passion for life with loving commitment to his family very well. We were forever filling in liberties that Time would concede. Andy was more important than a friend. I appreciated the newly weds lack of space, but they yielded uncomplainingly to the head-splitting demons that had plonked me on their sofa after another late night. I did not need mention my crumbled mental state because my one true lifeline with compassion was already there to lean on, and Andy didn't care whether I was demented, destroyed or drowned which was typical of the man.

Andy had enough bickering with university dropouts to keep him motivated in the University of London Union where he managed the odd cause célèbre (Ricky Gervais) in the printing offices. He was also up to the scary post-graduate society of his colleagues without blinking, although fresh blood was almost always being recruited for his Monday night quiz team. One demure statistic about Delius was never going to impress a soul, so we switched our attentions to another type of 'Sol', flavoured with a sprig of lemon. Our team was christened 'More Sols Than Sense' We were no more than a popgun among dashing infantry and the party smile shivering behind the sandbanks of a few sangrias was at its shyest. When I wasn't redeeming myself by answering straightforward wasn't redeeming myself by answering straightforward questions, my prattling insensibility was embarrassing. Once again I felt the mass murderer's blanket shield my eyes way from the intrusive strut of the assembly of judges who were doing no more than winding down the hard day's grind with a few beers. However I had to follow it through and enjoy competing on an equal billing with warm people I was surely never going to compete on an equal basis with for the remainder of my life, such was the chasm in our respective statures. I could otherwise be throwing myself from an eleventh floor balcony.

It should be said unequivocally that I was a complete nutter, although people have conflicting interpretations of one, when you are one. A nutter has likeable and unlikeable qualities which means that some more conservative elements are turned off by erratic form and some actually warm to it. My judgment was that the jury's acceptance of my behaviour was split down the middle, like I was. However, for nutters this is usually not enough, and this nutter in particular wanted to be loved by all. I shrank my bony ankles into my heels when I couldn't make others like me with missing friendly banter, which is funny and always popular. I had a wounded sense of humour, which I drew on to laugh distastefully at all my inner deformities like a spoilt child lunging at a cripple he has no wish to emulate. Laughter is the best antidote to pain, but it can't clean it out, and my maniacal high-spirits simply reinforced the lows because the more I failed with humour, the more disappointed I became with myself. My pain simply corrupted the higher innocence of laughter in its valueless shame. I was as determined to make people laugh as I was without wit. It was deuce and I could only consider my brilliance before when I was talented, sparklingly funny and popular without too much effort. Meanwhile a certain cause celebre (Ricky Gervais) was wasting his life in a ding-dong chess dredger with Andy between capturing a spellbound audience in the bars with a freakish one-man show that cracked more jokes open than the assembly of bottled beers lacing the alternative music dance floor. The crackling entertainment deserved a three-hour standing ovation but it pierced my tragedy because there were two Ricky Gervais's in the room, one sitting on Napoleon's throne and the other mutated with mental illness, sitting in the stalls, unable to contribute or share in the revelry. Like many of his guests I was unable to make the feeblest impression on his sweeping sense of humour, just sitting there compulsively, half in astonishment and half in jealousy. If I could make no amendments to his wit and that talented comedian could find no laughing panacea for my pain, then my downcast soul could only weep as it slowly sank down into the stodge. I was stretchered away from the show half giggling and half in agony.

It was this idolization of talent that had formerly been mine, and whose incarnation I could now only calculate which led me bumblingly to the film world and the agonies of mediocrity bestowed on Peter Shaffer's Salieri. After a year without work and all around me except Andy, questioning why I should throw away earning a crust for pallid trivia machine endowments, and no real hopes of any cessation in my ill-health, I recalled a genial reference made by Mark to the best film he had ever seen being 'Amadeus'. It was to be screened on Channel Four late one October night in 1990, where I confidently expected to retreat under the bed-covers of my old bedroom after a passable attempt to enjoy it. In a magical two-and-a-half hours of luxury however, the bed sheets were rolled untidily around my ankles. The film began with an old geriatric secured in an eighteenth century mental institution recounting his life story to an indisposed padre. The priest pompously asks the old man to confess his sins among them being the guilt behind the murder of Mozart, which is excused as caustic lunacy. To soften Salieri's temper, the Bible is reached for to give the same kind of peace I had reached for in my early days as a student. The holy man reads to the voice of experience so utterly desolate from his lifetime's journey - "All men are equal in God's eyes." Armed with real knowledge against a floppy paperback, Salieri tests out the soon to disintegrate priest with a quote from his own best source of literature, himself. "Are they?". The priest hastens his decapitation from authenticity when Salieri offers him the tragic involvement with Wolfgang Amadeus Mozart and his music, which seemed to be like hearing the very voice of God. And yet it was Salieri who had applied for Holy dispensation, labouring humility and chastity in return for a divine music that only he was able to recognize in the mawkish child of Mozart. As Salieri is forced to admit the mediocrity he didn't know he had, he vies jealously with his more imperious counterpart and turns finally against his Maker, the one he had trusted and who had abandoned him. The playwright, Peter Shaffer expressed the music into perfect words that befitted Mozart's status, and mine, and also the jousting horrors of Salieri's bitter defeat, which F.Murray Abraham acted so valiantly that I was turned show stoppingly mute by everyone's greatness. I sympathized with Shaffer's great musical dinosaur who was courteous and correct and yet incomplete without a scrap of the talent that God surely owed him. I warmed to the man who got thwarted by immortal genius and who vowed to get even with the architect of those flooded dreams; God Himself. I wanted to do that. To kill Mozart was to kill God, and as this justification dawns the confessional Bible waved so victoriously Salieri's lost cause, becomes a little greasy in the palm like the transparent illusion it has been trounced as. If God wrote a book of contradictory truths, then Shaffer wrote the absolute book of life and it was fitting for me that the unruly religion that had twisted me round its pernicious finger, should be dismissed unarguably as a cropper. That was what I wanted to know and after two-and-a-half hours I knew how it was logically possible to believe it. Even though the pain of my illness was still acutely insufferable, somebody, somewhere had got inside it, understood it and turned it on its head. And he had made God look like an arsehole in the process! Independently I will never be a great writer and Shaffer's Salieri will never be a great composer, but together we can recognize the incarnations of what we truly are, he as the composer and me as the librettist, and still truly be heard.

The religion that Shaffer shuffled into some consistent order for me was still pounding with God's intent to part the waters in the Waveney Terrace cabins, some eighteen months after my official departure. I still had no life to lose and scavenging from trivia machines in the London pub scene was so lonesome that it felt like being lost in the vast expanse of a national park. Scouring vacuous pubs was as trivial to the 'old me' as the machines I may not necessarily find bursting there with cash prizes. After buying my Capitalcard for three pounds, drinking watered-down coke, and purchasing lunch, I could expect to profiteer by a meager twenty quid per day for my investment, assuming my regular haunts had not been hunted down by quiz playing adversaries first. It was insanely melancholic and monotonous to exhaust myself, despite having the general knowledge of Old Father Time, but the facts were that I was unavoidably insane. The world I was in dictated its own rules of survival. If you couldn't find paid employment, then even if you were Bill Gates, in that condition you hustled like all the rest of the welfare wayfarers. However if this was practiced protocol for the new me, it was a standard short of a platitude for the old me. He still wanted desperately to go and see June as the April Wine she remembered him by, and not as the Meat Loaf slumped in gravy and sliced into slabs of cooking fat he felt had become. But instead of waving the white flag of surrender, he posted his tricolour courageously on enemy soil. How dare God smash one of the all-time great romances, blaming the innocent party for gutlessly walking off into the freedom of the wilderness, in debt, bloated and unhappy. Therefore, in a cosy pub in Greenwich after a smidgen of trivia remuneration, I assessed this émigré standing in an imposter's shoes and gave him a callous slap for not bucking the trend. I still had to cross the bridge of spies and explain to Junie how this beautiful young buccaneer had been reborn into old age without her knowing. What else could take my mind off the collision course other than the actual collision? I must try to find her in Wolverhampton or to whatever rock she had disappeared to. She would be too fickle to understand, but if I crossed the sagging bridge before it broke at least we wouldn't be standing on both divides of the abyss, never again to reach out our hands to hold and touch. I made an instant decision, which suddenly put me in the world of the BBC test card, and like the TV screen in the middle of the night I found myself in pitch-black darkness. I was surrounded by death and penetrated like ringworm. It was worse than a panic attack or stress because I was fully aware of my circumstances and alert. But all the lifeblood seemed to drain out of my veins like a gas pressure reading sinking on a barometer. It was like suffering a heart attack in the blurred frenzy of a concerned crowd you were leaving behind to pass on in to the after life from. Despite this anxiety, the world was still playing its jukebox as the children japed about in the beer-garden and the slippery trivia machine player in the corner gambled another unit. The trivia machine player in the corner was frozen cardboard. I pulled my scrambled senses together for a moment and revisited my slender window of opportunity. I hadn't died because I could see and feel my hands touching the buttons on the trivia machine, but I had come close and still might be as close; I didn't know. What I did know was that I had to return to Norwich and the multi-storey car park I could have jumped from two years ago, which was Waveney Terrace. God could still be forgiving if I followed the lifeline of His explicit instructions just once. Nobody would miss my subtle disappearance on a weekday and I had acquired enough train money for the well-fathomed two-hour route from Liverpool Street. If I could perform my task I could be home before Newsnight. I was tingling with the fear that I could be dead before each imprecise footfall hit the deck and I knew the odds of obeying God's saving auspices were slight after not having completed my mission in the less pressing days of relaxed revision, a whole month before my history degree was recorded. Even with the stakes being raised for my life I still felt strangely ambivalent and pessimistic for my safety. But I still had one last roll of the dice. In under four hours I would be standing in the huddled doorway of A Block, drawing on courageous stamina to change my life back to the real Rob as God had designated. I looked as dreadful as a mad prowler on the loose. No student could have guessed that I had spent three years there and lived in these same set of apartments. A couple of female students were already suspicious and put out feelers about a local man hanging around the porches at Waveney Terrace that should not be approached. As I flitted between Norwich guesthouses and emptied their trivia-machines to pay my way, the mucky rumours discouraged me from fulfilling my nemesis with each shriveling hour. Eventually I attracted some unwanted attention from residents who believed I was a Mr.-Hey-Look-It's-Only-A-Sausage fridge raider, and made some sarcastic requests to remove my frame and retrace my movements. While I hovered in the lobby a black student making a phone call threatened to thump me if I invaded his privacy again, but I was not paying any attention to his business. It was just one more nasty comment from a God who was supposed to be rescuing me. In the end however, I did take hold of the chaffing reins and with perspiring hands turned the handle on the next door to mine where the faint echo of graffiti still lay smudged from the Carboniser's previous reconnoiters. The room remained fastened and there was no superior flash of the divine. I was still not well and I hadn't been given a way out. My intuitive stab at bravery meant nothing. God may not have actually lied, because the plan had not quite been seen through to the letter, but I couldn't hang on further, and must take a trip back to London as a fallen angel of death. However, I flirted first with the sea-air of Great Yarmouth, which was under twenty minutes away by train, just in case God had any new ideas of protection. It was also a logical step for a traveler who needed respite.

 I rented accommodation nightly from a family B&B in the heart of thriving Yarmouth, and word had not carried to the lady proprietor that here was the mad prowler, that had been under feminist scrutiny in the lengthening shadows of the University of East Anglia seven days previously. Neither did she ask herself why a holidaymaker in the height of the summer season never strayed from his unmade bed, awaiting the swashbuckling will of the Holy Spirit. I was grateful that she didn't intrude on the respect of a licensee, because it might result in a blood sacrifice of a bed for a street to walk at night. I could only brave the party happening outside when I needed more cash prizes for my lodging and sandwiches, otherwise I was pole axed for days, listening to my only friend, the personal stereo, broadcasting the entire day's play at Wimbledon for a solid eight and a half hours on Radio Five. However cash flow problems meant the luxury of time was evaporating for this tiller of the soil and waterer of the well, and so I was moving on to the sandy beach in fine weather, looking so destitute that I wouldn't have minded if the tide had taken me out into the ocean. While I waited for the prodigal public to refill the coffers of the trivia machines I may just bear a few nights sleeping rough under the pier. I couldn't stomach seeing myself physically, but my darkened mood written on my once glowing cheeks, could have blended into the bathing background like any other destitute. However, in the bucket and spade daylight, a good Samaritan must have picked up on how I was presenting when he reached into his pocket and pulled out a whole five pound note. Among the dots of swimmers, he gave me more than a London street beggar will claim in a day, so I hesitate and shiver at my pitiful demeanour. Despite my predicament, I couldn't lax my principles and unbelievably refused this saintly offer, only for the man to press the money into my hand as if I was the most wretched person he had ever seen in his life.

There was a bowling alley among the amusement arcades and these were habitual sources of revenue for the trivia hunter. Instead of taking candy from a baby it was like taking pocket money from schoolchildren. Inside there was a bar and a cafeteria but no machine. Families were able to wander around the twenty-lane complex if they were on the waiting list for a game, and I staunchly but wearily observed them pouring money away on nothing more than crisps and cokes for treated youngsters like a careful yeoman. The Drifters were the top act for the seaside special and my decision to spread a little happiness with a great soul act that night was my last thought to connect with freedom. I don't know if it was due to the absence of one-armed bandits, but compared to the mists of children rolling oversized bowling balls down aisles that smacked the bunch of skittles disturbingly, the cafeteria was relatively threadbare. With some of my five-pound note, I could afford to buy a chicken curry and one drink. I collapsed my tray onto the iron rails while a waitress spooned some hefty yellow splodges onto my circular plate with some boiled rice, and then I spotted some fresh orange being poured from a tap into a plastic glass a few feet away by a customer further in front of me in the queue. I desperately needed vitamins and juice to filter down through my dry throat. However God deemed that I couldn't have one. Although I didn't have one, it felt like the final straw. I was too feeble in mind and body to obey any more commands and when my turn came I just released the tap to offload a waterfall of nutritious drink into my container. As the orange juice sprinkled down I felt a thudding sense of pain in the right hand wall of my chest. God had taken searing revenge very swiftly for daring to avoid His objectives. I visualized the pain like a white light from above so it was definitely the decisive punishment for my miscreance. In my student days I confidently hoped my heart would hold out for at least the stresses of my twenties, but as the pain spread westwards, I realized the foreboding heart attack was arriving much earlier than the biological forewarnings had protested. I sat into my table transfixed on the chest-pain like a musical statue at a children's party with my lukewarm plate of chicken curry uneaten by each item of unhandled cutlery. As the pain darted westward worryingly briskly, I fought tooth and nail to reconnect with a higher power of healing. The café was ghostily devoid of any matter except the musings and stirrings of the counter staff, which finally ended in an ambulance crew admitting themselves to the premises. I overheard one of the checkout girls mutter that they had been observing my posture for over three hours, but it would have been the same if it was twenty-five minutes. I was frozen with fear. The team assembled their kits and gave me an oxygen mask, which I palmed away from my nose and mouth every time God gave me specific instructions to obey Him. The team concluded that this erratic mechanism of non-survival was led by an attempted overdose. Searching for a solution that was not revealed, they injected me first with anti-drug medicine, before diagnosing heart failure. I was lifted onto a stretcher and carried out prostrate amid the impervious racket of skittledom with facemask, leads and all the accoutrements. The scariest point of non-redemption was when they had safely bundled me inside the hectic ambulance. I was literally losing consciousness when one of the uniformed depositors joked that there wasn't "much hope for this one." I didn't think I was going to die, but one still can't quite grasp this elusive reality even when one is at the finishing post. I tried to stay conscious during the ride to the general hospital by holding fast to the light of God and while almost comatose I flicked out my arms elastically in prayer to receive any particular order to avert the drastic conclusion. Strength of mind rallied with the strange optimistic belief that I could scramble out of this pit alive, and when the ambulance driver swung the vehicle through the iron gates, hope was stirring. Even with the attachments to my bare chest diagnosing the reality of the fall, my own driving willpower seemed to overcome what was clinically wrong with me. While I focused on God, I refused to let myself die, and I pulled determinedly on the deadly tightrope like an anchorman to a tug-o-war team. As they wheeled me into a ward on a trolley, I salvaged some consciousness and self-examined the chest pains which were decelerating at the rate they were inserted. I regained full awareness on the wooden hardboard bed surrounded by some exquisite looking nurses who were speechless after what they had just witnessed. I may have had a heart attack three hours ago, but I needed no life-saving surgeon to operate now, so amid grand astonishment I undid all the plastic leads and wires and threw myself from the stand as if they had rescued a hoaxer. This time span lasted no longer in my mind than it took Jim Kirk to leap through a vortex of another realm to storm another alien battleship. However I recall it with the clarity of a birth, somehow arriving in my mother's arms from a place I had no knowledge of. I don't know about babies but when I leant into the arms of a young and pretty nurse, she was having twins.

But seriously, when I crash-landed like Mr. Bean from the heavens, I fell straight away under observation like microscopic extra-terrestrial plant life. For one minute I was dying and the next I was assessed by the gathering entourage as a mild prankster. Standing modestly in just my black denim jeans, I was encircled like a hunted wild minotaur. The slightest lapse in concentration away from God's overview scared me to believe I would still certainly die from more imminent chest pains. The shame factor was actively employed to appease Him. I endeavoured to dance a ritualistic flagellation ceremony to wash away my reviled sins, and be of peaceful mind in God's good books. To be a vessel of His inner parenthood, He would accept sado-masochistic, medieval penitence, so I grabbed a young buxom nurse, and tried to do the most shameful thing I could think of and kiss her. This was my tithe. I kissed her unaggressively on her face, and followed this by trying to gently kiss her colleagues standing by. Security was ringside in a second, and 999 called to arrest an innocent disciple of Jesus who was being persecuted by the world that first hated Him. I was unaffected by the long arm of the law because the flaming power over me could still determine my immediate future, as it had done when I did drink from the cup of orange. The gawping nurses took pity on me while glancing eagerly over their shoulders for the blue-collar boys, and they sympathized with how sad it was to see this young lad so disturbed and agonized.

Two officers of the law crept up on this sad, disheveled wreck with due care and intention. The senior broker was quite stocky and shaven-headed. He was undoubtedly hardened to the day to day task of hauling in trouble makers, and he could see with all his experience that I was only tired and unwell, and not in the least bit criminally intimidating. The other cop was young and tall, and as silent as the grave had taught him to be. He also assessed that cajoling rather than coercion was the order of the day. The elder calmly iterated that they saw no necessity of arrest for the laughable show of indecency that the condemned lunatic had stirred up and the younger without seeming to open his mouth offered me the freedom of Yarmouth if I didn't return to annoy the neighbours. I couldn't answer and therefore didn't comply to their terms. They repeated their non-aggression pact several times before patience dimmed slightly and they deferred their tactics to the "other place" where "I really didn't want to go." They had given me options but they were already housed under the same thunderous sky that I had roamed indistinguishably under for five years of ill health. I still feared the loony bin as a place for dropouts and cocaine snorters, and I followed a divisively suspicious public trend toward them. If I had not been so tired and exhausted, I would have returned to the blissful communes of the bowling alley, but history could never be repeated like that. I just virtually gave up. I sank to my knees, and cupped my two hands behind my back (as God ordered) and waited for the cuffs, looking like an unfortunate oven-ready turkey. The stocky policeman confirmed that "he really wants to go there", so he slipped the handcuffs on loosely with the skill of a fencing instructor, prompting me urgently to the back-row seat of his blue and white panda car, parked adjacent to the hospital gates I was never going to see again. In the short hop to the sanatorium it was quiet enough to hear the midday nightingales sing. We arrived at breakneck speed just a few miles down the road from where it had all kicked off five years previously. It was still in me like the dark side of Paradise, without creation or elements, just biting suicide, which had lasted from confidence to desolation. I had circumnavigated no more than fifteen miles to reach that destiny.

As the patrol car limped up indifferently to the fortifications, the complex of huts lining the green turf like battle ramparts, reminded me of a prisoner of war camp with a smile on its face. The summer helped bathe the houses in a soft, tawny light. I still was reticent to move through the jungle's prying eyes and crammed my bulk into the furthermost corner of the leather upholstery, like a fly hiding in the cigarette ashtrays. The more elderly policeman asked me to gently attend the ward where arrangements had already been confirmed for my admittance. I shuddered without God's approval looking like a frightened rabbit. The officers resorted to muscle to save complexities. They lifted me from under the armpits and dragged me along the narrow, undesecrated footpath, through the swing double-doors, to a square cell where they hastily dropped me without my feet ever once touching the lino. The world and the Drifters were safe from my antics now, and I wasn't going anywhere unless I pegged out.

The hellish lifelessness froze my tongue. All around me I could hear the happy noises of patients, like children playing in the schoolyard. They seemed to be familiar with each other like they had been thrown like Christians and lions into the same arena. I feebly scraped on to the single bed, which was the only furnishing in my room. There was a solitary blinded window for light, which revealed nothing of the grounds round the hospital perimeters. The room was in shade, which dusted the blue, sunken walls like cages, and the floor was stone hard, like an old Norman cathedral. I was utterly without company, save for a plastic jug half-filled with tap water, and God who had stolen away the cup out of which to drink. There were no hanging pictures of sailing harbours, no shelves with books to read, no plants, no expense spared. I waited for fateful visitors, but the doctors were as visible as ghosts, and for thirty minutes I fended myself away from earthly temptations to be in God's empty providence. I feared more chest pains, and cushioned my expectant body by thrashing it up and down like a springboard to allay the blow of another seizure. I breathed in fitful gasps channeling the rhythm of my heaving chest at around fifty knots per second. It was the only method I knew to stay alive and even that seemed tenuous.

When the doctors turned the screw of the cold iron, door handle, my comforts were like a silent screen version of the Exorcist, with a torturer spinning the wheel of the rack, to splay my breaking bones in dissonant directions. I had been unaware for prior weeks that barely anything had been digested in my flattened belly, and that I was at the brink of starvation, when God had intercepted the chicken curry. The non-person whose eyes were rolling around in the back of his skull had forgotten what it had been like to be a person, and subsequently forgotten the methods of how to eat and drink. The chalice they brought to my lips, leaked straight out sideways onto the nave of the stony ground. A physical examination concluded that I had eaten nothing for three weeks and that I had to be forced to eat a healthy meal, before a detailed mental assessment could be deduced. As one of His meaningful attempts at a joke, God piled the voltage from the entire Christmas lights through my palsied body, asking me gently if I could take up my bed, which was fixed to the floor, and walk.

My mind disobeyed me and my body disobeyed my mind as the gang of logicians removed their clipboards from the apocalyptic room, deserting me to play table tennis with more functionable men and women. I was left supercharged if utterly broken for hours, with my mind concentrated on Him to allow me to disembark from the rack and greedily pour out a thimbleful of water. But no such chance! God was having such a glorious time!

Put yourself in the doctor's white coat. Here was a patient who was barely audible, and whose only piece of knowledge about the world was that he was trapped inside the mental hospital he had refrained from exploring for an expectant five years. No rescue could be performed, not even with a sedative pile driver. The staff therefore just abandoned me to my mental noxiousness. When the staring daylight faded through the happy window, a new aperture appeared about a foot square through the bolted steel door to provide the only source of electrical energy to my bedchamber. During my first night in the pound, I was observed wryly through this opening and closing slot, by black night nurses who would click back the harness to chuckle heartlessly at the quivering, naked sub-human, curled into a ball, clinging to air. One of them goaded another to "see this one" as she laughed rhetorically. Not all discrimination gets addressed in the safe NHS.

For the duration of my twenty-four hour wakefulness, I made nearly enough sips of water to clean my parched trachea. The only light in the cell was the whiteness of my eyeballs swimming around under my blonde curls like the oscillating heartbeat of two ping-pong balls. The commotion of a daytime mental hospital had been distilled by the commonplace with the hush and hum of the infra-red neon tubes. Quite a peaceful substitute. I had time to philosophize but there was nothing to question. There were no whys or whens or ifs and buts. I was just there and it required no explaining. I was not tearful enough for an innocent victim passing through the eye of a storm, because I was quite utterly blocked. The unspilled tears that I wanted and needed to cry simply stoked up more pain of mental illness.

With the rising of the early wanderers to the creaking breakfast trolley that squeaked along the vestibules, came a renowned Persian psychiatrist who crept around my bunker with vivid horror. He was astute enough to realize that I was beyond the immunity of analysis. There were no consolations, not even a 'good morning, how are you?' He simply stroked the palm of my right hand between his thumb and forefinger like I was his own child. It was the best and only treatment. Instead of the angry flash of the Lord's healing, it had come down to this and it landed freely and without shaming my self-attitude. He left and returned throughout my first morning, straddling through the unhappy religious mania and the communication worthy of a dead horse, to administer orange squash, which freed me from the foreboding insult I had leveled at God in the bowling alley. Every logical movement in my brain was cancelled in triplicate by God, but when I saw the matter-of-fact doctors and nurses going about their business, I ascertained that there existed protection from the excessive punishments for religious blasphemy. I didn't have much to say to my personal helper when he collected me in a wheelchair for lunch. I was hungry but mental diminishment chewed my appetite up and spat it out like the rawness of hospital food. When I was fed a Brussels sprout cycling round a tablespoon, I took a bite and it tasted like a marvelous vitamin nutrient, like it was the ice-cold lemonade I desired on this one particular Summer afternoon. The three I did consume were as natural as an orchard full of succulent apples, or even the call of a blackbird. As I slumped forwards unstrapped from the wheelchair, I was led like a pet lamb back to my freshened room, where I collapsed on the stone cold paving, perhaps not like a trembling rabbit, but as a petrified, stone-dead dodo.

It may have been a couple more weeks before they followed up on my next of kin, and although I had not lifted my leathered tongue to speak, I had been bathed by two male nurses and shaven off the ginger growth beneath my chin that Catweazle would have been proud of. I was lucky to have family and friends who I unarrogantly knew would be sure to check up on what they had not recorded to be going on. They would also view an uncoordinated vegetable, unable to walk or talk and that would surely be nothing to boast about. It would be more scarring than a cohort of male nurses stripping you naked and scrubbing your private parts down untenderly with a crusty sponge, as if they were cheap hairdressers sweeping up the clippings of the day's head of hair. Being wheeled around the hospital for a few minutes by my attendants was a more of a curious luxury for me than the other carefree patients. Through catatonic eyes I was able to determine a modern hyper activeness under the bungalow roof that spread out into double single sex wards, recreational facilities, and TV screens dotted everywhere like night watchmen. I motioned to the handlers that I wasn't going to slip out unnoticed if they parked in front of the two television screens buried high into the thick-whitewashed plaster outside my bedroom, and they agreed to leave and go about their daily business. Had I been in London I would have tuned into the British Open golf event of 1991 anyway, but by happy fortune I could alternate my armchair spectatorship with the undiscovered pathways of satellite channels and MTV. With rock music still maligned as the 'devil's music' and 'evil', I could have had another seizure to learn that Bryan Adams' classic ballad, 'Everything I do (I

Do It For You), was at Number One, venturing on to be the most successful single of all time. Possessing a couple of well spun Adams' discs in my record collection made it sweeter, because his recording career seemed to have undeservedly nosedived since his peak in the mid-eighties. 'Everything I do (I Do It For You)' was number one for the exact same length of time I spent on the ward. No more and no less, but I saw no significance in that.

I also saw no significance when I was wheeled in under ten blankets to a side-door office, too jaded to make protestations with a bearded male nurse who was brandishing a hypodermic like a pneumatic drill. I made no objections when my full-time helper got me to stand, releasing my leather belt, enabling my smelly black jeans to fall to the ground. All was in line with the Great Yarmouth Convention. I was still disorientated by my surroundings and still numb to the rule book being thrown at me when the injection was slammed into my thigh muscle. My key-worker diverted my slept-in jeans to my waist again and I was invited to recline in my chair, while my middle-aged assailant tore into his files of match statistics with the precision of Eric Bristow, without motioning us to leave. I had no clue that I had just made dense contact with the helping hand of Section 3 of the Mental Health Act 1893, which submitted that a patient who was a danger to himself or others could not refuse treatment by law. A gallon of Clopixol was my treatment. The world was just as insane as I was and I couldn't argue with insanity from a position of insanity, because the product of insanities does not make sanity.

Gradually I took the commanding step of washing my own body while the clinical entourage observed the crusty sponge being applied to my naked manhood from behind the frames of their dark clipboards, and I squandered the naivety of the child bathing in proud inviolability by its mother. In return I felt the testing bashfulness of a retired geriatric being rendered helpless by its learned overseer. I was encouraged by the empiricism of my key-worker to admit the fork to my mouth at mealtimes and dissect the boiled Brussels sprouts that were my energy with my knife. The force of such rigour was soon somberly overtaken by a sleeping daze, which was too heavy to lift my stiffened legs into action. My dormancy lurked in the lengthening summer shadows, making the evenings shorter when the hours of remission should have been longer. But there was so little to occupy myself, that crashing out completely on my bed was my only hobby.

The dimensions of shape and colour were beginning to assemble around the flag of skull and crossbones I was waving. My single room was airy and as safe as any cathedral. The sun shone daily transforming the dusty grey walls into a pale, delicate unobtrusiveness that warmed me. An outstretched palm of thanksgiving so desperately fought with to relinquish one solitary drink, restocked the jug of water I had daily and I lurched to it and from it without reproach from the Lord. I developed a third twin relationship with the brotherly telescreens in the lobby, and it was probably felt that I was detoxicating myself from preoccupied stalemate with God to flooding intoxication with Bryan Adams on MTV and the golf which I lingered on through from Rice Krispies until Brussels sprouts. I still felt morbidly afraid of sinning and welcoming God's unimaginable fiendishness, but enjoying the sport in a lobby free from traffic was like relaxing in a Chesterfield, somewhere in Chesterfield, while reaching for the Times crossword and slurping a slow Pimms. There were few interruptions from the screaming suicidals I had fictitiously imagined and most people sailing beneath my bridge of spies were average folk, clean and personable, almost as if they were respecting another man's one-minute of silence. My lobby was a codeful of etiquette where I was left in peace and splendour to marvel at the dove-white ceilings and the three armchairs looking on to the narrow vestibules meandering down to the full day hospital circus, without ever once glancing back down the aisles over its shoulder. My invention is dreamy, but it became a necessity.

I was still listening through the motions of MTV overkill when my first shocked visitors greeted me. I possessed no driver's license or credit cards but the administrators had shuffled all sorts of forms to locate my next of kin. When both parents arrived, the mortal anguish renewed itself through embarrassment with God tightening up my swelling top shirt button. I instantly gave way to the cadaverous shell. They had turned over to a blank page when they saw the by-product of five years of unrelenting hell that I already knew. The tank load of Clopixol fixed the joints of my mouth together and when I tried to speak, I simply dribbled down the corners of my flushy face. I couldn't decipher their immediate reaction because reading human response was out of the question in my condition. All that was said went above me. God was having a good time though and finding all this a colossal gas. I felt wearied by His backstabbing, but I still figured that to appease His anger at my frailty was the only way the madness was going to get resolved. I was so convinced of my one-way impending doom, I invented some God-speak to my father to attain the services of a minister in Mount Sermon church in the backwaters of Norwich. He could perform the ceremony of last rites perhaps better than that of a last supper. My father would have obeyed any wish of mine, particularly a dying wish, while my mother anxiously trudged off behind him to track down this man of God. They locked themselves away in a Yarmouth B&B for the weekend after the nagging three hour drive from London and saw such little progression in their son's movements that they must have wondered if he would ever leave his hospital chair. However with every pounding the Clopixol walloped me with, I began to stretch out and doze in my cell again to suggest I wasn't utterly frozen solid. Occasionally the nice psychiatrist would make unreciprocated conversation, but he eventually yielded to the yet kinder auspices of the minister who had driven down specially to confirm a stray blasphemer's faith in Christ. The doctor gave way to my wishes and hoped for the best. When the young minister dazzled through the steel-rimmed doorway, the room became surly again, the jug of water was a poisoned chalice and I was thrashing my back around on my spring bed like a pop-up doll. The doctors parted company for my spiritual regeneration. I wouldn't talk to the minister who laid his palms gently on my head as he tried to perform an exorcism. Suddenly it became clear in my horrendous nightmare, that he was cranky, and that I was the victim of another of God's vicious jokes. Why was God mocking me? Why was God taunting me? I was insane, schizophrenic, suicidal, depressed, broken-hearted and cracked up and now this. God's holy orders were now trying to convince me I was possessed by some sort of evil spirit, which didn't fit, into my rounded thinking. I had swapped the gentlemanly hand-holding of a trained practitioner for an aggressive, outdated, snobbish and life-hating religion which regarded my helplessness as evil. Never again would I ask for God's intervention, for all I had ever got were crimes against my already diseased person. Soon God's agent was terrifying me by trying to cast out demons a la Jesus, which I knew simply didn't exist. It was the lowest point of my entire history. The religious Judas conceded defeat finally and went back to his flock on greener pastures with even the medical profession sizing him up after his bizarre, ethereal diagnosis. The kind doctor was so lost for words that he even quizzed me about demon possession. Nobody knew me or how to attend to my inner turmoil.

My trusted friends were soon on the spot to support me more capably. Andy and Simon were resolute but unsurprisingly shocked by their sporty, confident and educated school buddy looking like the Mummy, swathed under a couple of hundred blankets, but I couldn't hide my true spirits which had devolved from the fear of the sinful nature of conversation. I communicated with Andy better than most when I could because both still perceived a sense of humour about even a tidal wave of tragedy. Simon already knew too much with a perception way above the doctors, not so much work-related but friend-related. He could see what was going on from the start but waived his expertise for pure friendship. The key to my convalescence was the unceasing support of these friends and family and not the hit and run shock tactics of the vicar. Most patients had nothing like this and it was possible they would never come to terms with their illnesses. While all was fairly black and white, the pale blue washed walls began to paint themselves in a thin glow, and I received a massive boost from Denz who made an unexpected phone-call out of the royal blue. Like many who knew me, when we spoke, he couldn't hide his sympathy at the so-called deterioration and the depression in my voice; and so he told me. He was there and would surrender all work commitments to the cause which I turned down, redeeming my doyen of politeness again. However his genuine concern was noted like he had told me who won the two hundred metre backstroke for men at the Antwerp Olympics. I told him that a visit was not merited on this particular invalid. Denzil was probably shell-shocked with just words rather than pictures to inform him, but what my actual visitors believed about their shrinking elephant hardly necessitates print.

My vitality and not my fitful madness was the first to gather ground in those first few epidemic weeks. I became conscious of the wards I was pacing up and down in despite the catatonic haze of injections they were shooting me up with. I still owned the same gentle-giant of a key-worker who had pulled out all the stops to arrive at the newsagents across the road for confectionery every morning to break up the monotony of shoving Brussels sprouts through my guard and into my face. Early signs of recuperation were also evident when I got bored expecting visitors to arrive. Having been admitted to the ward amid a frenzy of fuzz, the other patients were still pretty much incognito, and I retreated into my own auspices. The buckets of Clopixol made me walking dead, which magnified the living death of my illness, for all my visitors to worry about. The doctors had fresh hope in this renewal however, and bought me a ticket to the luxurious 'ECT Suite'. This cunning simile simply means let's watch Prisoner Cellblock H, and was employed during phase one of the 1389 Mental Health Act. This rest-room held as much terror for me as Winston Smith's Room 101. I did know what the score was. They would knock me out with an anesthetic before slapping on the electrodes to grind four thousand volts of electric current through my temples. I understood that no other system of care could be more archaic. The debate for me however, was not the pointlessness of ECT but the massive fear of general anesthesia. Only supreme efforts of concentration on God had enabled me to beat heart failure and now this form of semi-consciousness was about to be blinded. Without this one thread of life, I would be killed mentally and unable to sustain my engine like a car failing its MOT. If the lights went out on my conscious brain, wouldn't an electrical energy field finish it off? Was this God's final masterstroke? This 'ETC Suite' became a showcase of terror and unnatural habitat, and to forcibly treat me they had to pin me down like some mad medieval monarch.

I woke up from my nightmarish adventure nearly two hours later with a soft pillow beneath my head, which was throbbing a little after the five-minute induction of light waves connecting my temples. After a cup of tea and two rich tea fingers I was alive and free, despite there being absolutely no miraculous transformation to my mental state. No surprises there. The only shock to my system was that hell was simply a deeply poignant reality. Nobody had told me what they were trying to achieve with this or the injections, and why it actually made me feel worse. However, unlike the injections the harm done was purely psychological and I walked free to explore the rest of hospital home-comforts. When I could dress, wash and eat by myself, I was offered some cooking experience in the large occupational therapy workshop, two doors down the left aisle from the lobby, where I sauntered past two more private TV lounges. I was instructed on how to cook shortbread, and pleased with my efforts I hid it under an old newspaper beneath my unmade bed to protect it from hungry night-thieves who were everywhere. After two hours only half remained and I had not eaten one, but it broke the sad conferment of stalemate into a moment of sour amusement and it did save me from eating them. Perhaps the wall of fear could not be broken by hysterics, but a sense of humour at the utterly ridiculous always helps. I wanted to go home now. I couldn't avoid the life that had so troubled me, but I didn't want to be under lock and key, wading through the same deep waters in a safe-house. After two more months of sitting on my Clopixol filled arse I was discharged, and Bryan Adams was no longer at Number One.

9

To dot the the I's and cross the eyes I was beaten off with a coach load of catatonic Clopixol which ensconced me in the Land of Nod for two solid months thereafter. There was no inaneness or trips to faraway planets afforded by illicit medications: this was as crushing as a sledgehammer to a walnut. My G.P attributed this phrase to my mother, but she said there was no other option than to pioneer a dose ready to knock out ten strong horses. With the ship temporarily steadied, my parents hired a seaside chalet in Mundesley, a beauty spot on the Norfolk coast, where I could shed the nine to five institutionalization of July and August. Andy kindly attended for moral support with his wife pregnant and the best chance in years to bury my golf game. Andy, forever the initiator of the tour itinerary, fixed up the snooker, table tennis, bowls and golf, while my parents rested with furrowed brows, taking scenic walks along the crescented bay. The tranquility of empty lanes replaced the deafening noise of an all-systems-go holiday town, with twittering old-age pensioners, and the melancholic homilies of fishing trawlers proudly honking off their captures. It was not enough for me because I was quite suicidal and nothing, not even an exorcism, could reframe my mental state. It began to slowly click that it was the daylight raids on the hospital drugstore that was completely zonking me. If I wasn't tucked up in bed before the sun went over, I would surely fall asleep in my dinner plate, as eggs are eggs. I would be lucky to welcome only six full hours of daylight, when I arose at half past eleven in the morning, and sit through the day, tired, sluggish and lethargic. The worst physical hell was the walking and even the local village pub seemed a marathon distance, which the town planner had situated craftily for our tour planner to slip away to with my father to discuss agenda. My legs were as stiff as an ironing board and would have been discarded by Douglas Bader for his preferred prosthetic limbs. Each time I paced out a foot ahead it felt like I was lumbering a hundredweight on each leg. There was so little action in my joints and limbs that I was shot to pieces above the neck and paralyzed from the waist down. I was unconscious both in the many hours of sleep and in the wakeful routine of the day, all in the gloriously untested name of anti-psychotic medication. Taking a swamp load of Clopixol was like conferring the latest torture gadget on a victim who had already crashed sonically through the pain threshold of death. It was simply another illness to fight illness with, and therefore it doubled rather than alleviated my suffering. I was like a blind man staggering across a Formula One circuit, and anyone with a bean of common sense including my mother could see it was killing me. Arrangements were installed to see the parish practitioner who at once prescribed a side-effects tranquilizer called Procyclidine. He was aghast that the proper mental health doctors had not supplied this on discharge. As soon as I took them, there was such a marked improvement that the following morning I allowed Andy to take me apart on the golf course which measured over 6000 yards in walking distance excluding hooks and slices. When the bottle of Procyclidine tablets had been emptied, I was behaving normally and handling the holiday like a champion walnut.

The relay races all over London to find trivia machines were still my only remittance. I had no capacity for work and felt ashamed to collect the unclaimed benefits I truly deserved. Therefore for the next nine months I relied on the goodwill of my parents, and my life in Hell continued. I was still being fed medication at home, although it was formally decided to acquaint myself with Clopixol's slightly less psychotic younger brother, Depixol which was more like the constant tapping of a twelve foot sledgehammer. The new drug made me drink and eat forever and my flamboyant lifestyle up at the University of London quiz nights and general town painting bloated me like Henry VIII. I slipped down the snake pit of self-esteem easily with no ladder to regroup. Jesus was still ordering me to be or not to be and I was becoming dangerously compulsive when activated by His gracious instructions. However when I employed the defensive strategy of 'Amadeus' its intellectual reasoning parried God's frantic lunges and He became more desperate. I wasn't just watching the film I was constantly learning about life from it. Salieri's accusations leveled against God's injustice were fair and as reasonable as my own. I sympathized with the way God had humiliated the character not just with music if that wasn't derisory enough, but with cocky home-truths and indelicacies which struck at the heart of a really good man. I could never believe the admonishing critics rampantly accusing Salieri of the jealous murder of Mozart, he had simply been pushed far too far over the brink by a jealous God. And that was as indisputable as my whole life story. Antonio Salieri was my bitter riposte against a Betrayer who in my bleakest and darkest hour had mocked me with Mozart's Masonic giggling. I wasn't delirious about Christianity any more. I knew it, Salieri knew it, and God "forced to listen".

Paying for my upkeep was lost to the trivia-playing veteran and my absent support team that should have followed up in after-care. My splintered legs couldn't stroll around the great city as before and the utter despair at being unemployable at twenty-four in a family of accredited achievers really began to whack me. I took bar work and was so faltering that one man-

manager sacked me after a single shift. I worked for peanuts in my father's local also, but before 9pm it was noticeable of how ill I looked to the drinkers. It was embarrassing trying to be a friendly custodian with good manners and hospitable when my frowning expression was like a satanic expletive. It was not inviting to paying customers who had escaped for the evening from precisely this. When my flabby fingers could not even fit inside an empty drinking glass to clean it I handed in my notice. My situation was dissolving with no opportunities, no talent, no hope, and no social services.

The only job interview I passed was when I was the only candidate, and that was mighty close. When I was offered this chance to work in a TV rental outlet in Forest Hill less than a mile away, I believed that fortune had for once smiled on me. The shop opened at 9am and was an easy deadline for those not struggling with Depixol oversleep. Each morning I had the munchies and before I called in next door to work, I zestlessly slumped over the McDonald's counter and tamed my hunger with the fry up I had been waiting all night long for. For a computerphobe the work duties were not taxing, but the inter-personal relationships were hazardous to build up, not least because the other two staff were convivial and damn good at their jobs. However, even with straining to keep up with the gossipy banter my colleagues were equal to the task of accepting me at face value, which was all they could do. Anything less and they would have decided enough was enough and thrown me to the lions. Not least were they sharing people and they made me feel wanted. The earnings softened the blow of yuletide, and the yelping cries in my mind over what I was going to do to keep everybody happy, but I was still on show and unable to blend into the background among customers who wanted attractive salesmanship. One day in the New Year of 1992 I flipped at the prospect of another vigorous nine to five, like I was going down a mineshaft. The mental illness was the prominent factor, but the other illness of medication made me feel at eight o'clock in the morning, like a lame horse running over fences in the four and a half mile course at Aintree. I didn't fancy it, and I had earned enough requisite pay to fuel my blood flow.

That day I dressed for work in my undersized uniform and bade farewell to my folks and headed for the January sales where I spent enough time nosing around to confirm my story, before returning home for dinner at 6pm. When I peaked around the kitchen door, they all knew I hadn't been working. My father headed the investigation and spoke cautiously. He said, "the manager rang..", and by that time I was already weeping. I bombed out of the kitchen up the hall stairs and along the landing to my bed to sleep off the drug for yet another insanely early night. When morning broke I fastened myself to my duvet unable to face anymore. The following day I was still there and my local G.P and a social worker were called in. I spoke no words with my tongue on an elastic string, glued to the carpet. I was interrogated for some minutes and although I comprehended every single question, I simply had nothing left to answer for. Finally when the G.P sat me up with a mug of tea, I released some in-depth paranoia, which she quite justifiably reviewed as rambling psychosis. I wasn't dragged in off the streets to the local psychiatric hospital which I never knew existed in downtown Hither Green, I was hauled in with the dignity of a laird being shown the red carpet for his chariot. Nevertheless I was in again and my days were numerical.

Less than two miles from home, and sixty seconds from Andy's place, Hither Green Hospital was an overbearing late Victorian style prison that resembled the Addams family estate. It was so decadent that only two psychiatric wards were functionable in a complex seven times as great as Yarmouth. Many psychiatric patients who see ghosts probably first saw a headless green knight in the grounds of Hither Green. In Great Yarmouth the floor space was the domain of the people to circulate and entertain in; in Hither Green, there was one stuffy and oppressive corridor to pace off the miles of unsettling medication. The grounds, however were not without historic charm and one could conceptualize the late Victorians gathering there to walk off the healing spa waters along the myriad pathways they had left behind.

When my name was recorded in the register, I was shown to my cubicle with just a shower curtain ringlet between the next guy and me, but before we were properly introduced, my trousers were around my ankles and I was snorting another dose of Depixol from the wrong end again. Alexandra Ward was never what I would call stereotypical chaos. The nurses judged most people as being too ill if they didn't circulate for their 8am bowl of Rice Krispies, when in truth they were completely pie-eyed from the mountains of injections prescribed. The people lay in state along the one corridor of twenty four cubicles, and rose only from the peace and quiet of their snoring to the antiquarian TV and radio which each may not last the day's internment. In the office the nurses viewed their cherished ones over their lunchtime menus, and the more enlightened of them would leave it to the friendly student nurses to pace up and down with the patients to the bathroom at the neck of the corridor and the locked gates at its shoulder. This was a London hospital that catered for twenty three thousand inner city residents where mental illness was spreading like flu. I imagine that the reason it couldn't hold a candle to Great Yarmouth was because the powers that be didn't care if it worked or not. If they had they would have managed space less nefariously

Hither Green was thus boring and depressing and a third minor illness to contend with, but I was not in there without reason. Everybody now knew I was ill, but my family was still my most familiar visitors. Their one hour stop-bys between five and six were the only source of light to penetrate the stone brickwork and the feeble red curtains cutting us off from the high, bolted windows. Jesus and God were tripping unopposed through the manifold swamps of my mind again like outlaws, lassoing every thought and dream, impeaching them and then sending them off to the funeral pyres as heretics. Consequently there were moments when I disregarded my father, mother and sister, and then speak impeccably to a staff nurse at two o'clock in the morning if He so desired. By now the physical stress was controlling my behaviour like a fourth and climactic illness. My system was overheating with no energy left to conserve, and I was already refusing food, drink and sleep to appease God. The medication illness was bloating my body up like a pressure cooker needing a lid and my internal organs were dancing around the earth's orbit, or simply ready to fail and die. The mental exhaustion was immense. Every time I spoke of these symptoms to a duty nurse, after the lunchtime menu had been sorted, she would return with a brand new hypodermic needle to calm me down. I was lazily intuitive still to know that if I confessed to a nurse or a doctor in confidence, I might soon be dead. One day I carried the notion that if I remained seated in a particularly gross living room chair, God would not be able to kill me. I was so paranoid about His condemnation, that I believed even the slightest fidget would result in the end. I believed I was safer during mealtimes, which were delivered to my throne by hand, and I was still safe during Newsnight. I remained awake, alert and safe until next morning, but the stress required concentrating on safety for sleepless days made death almost inevitable in my unhygienic state. I spurned my right to shave and wash down my ghastly features with freshening soap, and I rejected the five-yard trip over to the 9am breakfast trolley with the world and his wife spilling the contents of the milk jug over three-inch diameter cornflake bowls. I was in this chair to stay for expiration and I only communicated with a nod or shake of the head. It was Doomsday.

The afternoon entertainment was the 1992 European Championship football final between Denmark and Germany and a posse of sedated wildcats had gathered mournfully in front of the interference on TV. I had not slept for forty-eight hours, but was looking forward to the game myself. With the Danes winning one-nil, my mother appeared over my shoulder and sat by me tenderly. Neither of us spoke, probably inviting the other to begin the preliminaries. This was it. I got a clearance sensation in my pickled forest of dissonance, and without due cause I was reunited with my sanity. In that split second or two I was the full ticket. I looked at my calm, kind mother in her eye like no time ever before and purred unstutteringly, "Mum. I'm better." Mum was unmoved by commonplace sensationalism. Jadedly, if a little hopefully, she replied, "are you?". And I just said, "Yes".

AND THE RECOVERY

10

When I was ill God mocked me; when I was well God persecuted me. The recovery from this nauseating madness was very far from instantaneous. Even on this day as I write well nearly two years after the twin towers massacre of September 11, my own cut-throat war is raging for the peace, the bombers seemed to destroy so unamicably. Now my spirit droops like an over lagging branch ready to be chain sawed, before the next and latest admiring gardener will be confounded by my outpouring of spring blossom. This island of survival is however bolstered by the great stubborn tree trunk made of great British oak. I won't deny that this past decade has been as fortunate as it was virulent. I saw the disfigurement every day like a late Sunday afternoon in summer and I collected a bloom of olive boughs from the dusty wasteland, but I conclude that I cashed in my readies for a set of angel's wings and a harp.

I have just made a jug of morning coffee in my percolator, which I secured for twenty pounds on a bargain hunt in Croydon. I reflect that I am thankful to not need to serve my spending habits by reconnoitering the old haunts on the London underground map where the clinkity-clunk of trivia machines now sit unemployed in silence. I reflect that lately I am never panicked into drinking too much by my illness. If I was assigned a photographic project from the classes, I would click my brand newish second hand pocket camera to include the naturally peaceful environment of the coffee maker because nested on the kitchen shelves behind it are not dishes, but a treasure-trove of signed celebrity 'stills' which I value highly, even more than the fridge-freezer I have not cleaned properly since my mother deposited the money for it some six months ago. The kitchen is not strictly-speaking for visitors, but I am not lazy and if I want to create a good impression, I wave them through to the centre of the universe to recline on my Chesterfield and survey the formidably scary Austin Powers relics and all my other celebrity snapshots which now include an enigmatic Carol Decker and Frankie Dettori lookalike, Ben Elton (without his specs on). I afford a satisfied intake of breath around this sitting room that has become a masterpiece of invention for the past eight years or so. Michelle ordered me to trust her when she redesigned the mottled yellow walls to an unsubtle green flicker, which she borrowed from her hair pattern once seen down Carnaby Street as she swayed to the swinging rhythm of Marc Almond on her headphones. I always trusted Mad Michelle when she had an intellectual instinct, but looking at the backdrop of the clear blue sky filled with a radiant Sun through the blinded window, to a backdrop of dusty lime green paintwork, I shall wonder if this was one of her better moments. However this cool intellectual glow offsetting the beating hot June sunshine could not have been inspired by anybody else, and I reminisce about the mountains of fag butts and stale mugs of instant coffee she left behind to haunt my sitting room before it had any kind of character. I could never have survived in the loneliness that independent living arranges without my CDs, which I spin religiously at moderate volume to protect my secretive neighbours below. I still do not drive despite making detailed noises to the contrary, but I am able to transport stereo systems for a quarter of their value from Hayes, near Bromley, by cab from the money that I save by not being on the roads. Work that one out! Just how important the CD player has been overall will be highlighted hitherto.

As I sip from my Chris Rea tour mug, which I acquired in

Sheffield last year my gaze wanders around the four rooms of this comfortable flat that is my self-made home. I see that I have a fascination with grown-up toys, particularly the delights of Elvis Presley memorabilia. When my phone rings from behind the line of the seventies cocktail bar, a statuette of the great man starts shaking his hips to the ring tone of 'Jailhouse Rock'. After seven thousand rings, this becomes far from idyllic because I am only a moderate fan of this song and the early part of his career. Treason. Friends tell me my nest of home comforts say much about me. I would state that if it does then it is because it is tacky but not a disgrace. The more alarming extrovertness of the place is reigned in by a basic TV and computer, and an ordinary gas fire, which has an Eiffel Tower miniature sitting aloft for an unannounced reason. Oh well. These amenities are used sparingly, although the TV is used despairingly, and that's not a joke. The other night Andy phoned me up on the king's phone to tell me exhaustively that he had come close to 'groining' the TV screen after England's diabolical victory over Slovakia in midweek. I would do this if I had less patience with the current crop of BBC sitcoms, and presenters who relinquish their plumy Oxbridge accents for the working man's language of the North. Some presenters try three accents at the same time. George Orwell they are not. Except when I replay a favourite American film on video, television writers, and especially so-called British comedy writers, make me fell sad and bemused that I could have once outgunned them and exalted the genre. I was awakened in the seventies to the creative cream of British comedies all unharnessed by political intervention when funny was funny. In the golden era of my childhood, my mother could not drag me from the half-inch gap between myself and the TV screen, from the custard pies of Saturday morning 'Tiswas' to the burly thrills and spills of 'The Professionals'. Who could blame a child who was being properly educated by what he viewed? My favourite seventies sitcom which even pulped the might of Dad's Army and the genius of Fawlty Towers was It Ain't 'Alf Hot Mum. Even the title I find amusing, because with the exception of Mr 'La Di Da' Gunner Graham, the concert party were the sort of innocent striplings who would write such unsoldierly notes home to mother. And such feebleness in the line of duty I could relate to. The reason this masterpiece can never be repeated is because it was too honest about stereotypes; there is no avoiding that the best comedy always is, if it's funny. However in a town hall society of comic indifference to race, sex and gender unless you're black, gay or female, the most politically sound TV sitcoms of today will fail, simply because the funny bits are excerpted. Yes Minister for example, succeeded because it was still politically unsound. That well-known bright spark, Tony Blair would have hated it, so it must have been hilarious. Perched on a picture hook overlooking the Scooby Doo biscuit barrel that rests on a coffee table on stilts that Dave generously parted company with just for me is a portrait of Martin Luther King who interests me marginally less than the original Martin Luther. The message of peaceful petitioning favoured by that other hero, Ghandi is of personal fascination to me, but nobody can argue that these men lacked a sense of humour. As a British man I can laugh at the grotesque indictment of British and Asian culture endorsed by Goodness Gracious Me. Could not Ghandi have found the grotesque indictment of British and Asian culture made by It Ain't 'Alf Hot Mum equally as funny? If only he had been Director-General of the laughably unfunny BBC.

It is with considerable regret that these non-toleration methods are exacted by a Health Service that has discharged me haphazardly from its care. My mother says it is an important step for me because it reveals how much ground I have covered with a schizophrenic disease, and I do trust her judgment even further than Mad Michelle's. I am still just about permitted to attend the Sydenham drop-in centre for mental health, if I do need help which since the early days has been vastly supportive. Staff welfare now rules our services, which are in need of a hearing aid. The all out assault on public condemnation of mental illness has replaced the healing of the sick which is all very commendable, but hardly necessary. When I first met Michelle in 1997 on a drama course, I discovered the unpressing urgency for a non-committal society to even care about mental illness. Both of us had decided to restructure our lives by studying drama, despite coming from domestic opposites in life, yet we were firm about who we were and also about each other. If I had handed one of the Trust's leaflets on prejudice she would have shot me. Why? Because she wasn't prejudiced. The Trust would have argued rather hypothetically that by doing something work-related I was escaping the jaws of institutionalization, but my key-worker, Barry, quite rightly concluded that by doing this course I was engaging in a risk. This assessment was born out after one day when I thought about killing myself such was the pressure. According to the Trust there are no limitations to mental illness, but Barry and myself would argue that it depends on where you are with it. Initially I was scared to introduce myself to the class without disclosing my schizophrenia, although the teaching staff all knew and were forgiving because the acting skills I had perfected at UEA could now be imparted before other students. If I could put suspicious minds off the scent in my own back yard then I should know about leaping into another character easily. So despite a brilliant actor and having a perky memory for trivia, the learning of lines could not have been more terror-filled. In the four anxious months I attended before dropping out with nervous exhaustion, I was filmed being struck dumb by stage fright, trying to invent new lines for 16th century English tragedy, and quarrelling with a very insistent voice coach that speaking like Joan Greenwood was unnecessary. My line about Don Henderson cut no ice either, although Michelle loved it. Gladly, she could entertain the ridiculous. Barry was always intuitive with advice but the huge risk did contrive to find a friend whose broadminded perspective on the truth could not victimize those it had deceived. She knew I was ill and I knew her mind was hyperactive. We both bore our crosses intellectually with her fast tongue and my fast brain. We never accepted anybody on the surface because of our Freudian curiosities, which dealt a hammer blow to any type of bullshit wafting over. When she observed me she was not in the least bit sizing me up a deranged lunatic the Trust was preparing me to be judged as, but as a complete and rounded individual she adored. This made both her and I feel better than a leaflet campaign to patent the world's condemnation of mental illness. In fact life took care of us, so I at least began to realize that prejudice in any shape or form is what you make it. Through the power of one insightful mind and a bit of good luck I was able to never walk around under a schizophrenic cloud again. It never ceases to amaze me what life is out there and that prickly word itself, I view as no more than a media invention to mislead us. Schizophrenia doesn't even describe half of me, and if it does, then both of us are entirely misunderstood. I haven't seen Michelle for some years now since she moved to Nottingham, but somehow I still wish she could be privy to the Hazel Irvine picture, the leopard skin bedspread, and the dolphins on my toilet seat, that she did not witness first time round. However there might still be time for my sitting room to be redeveloped with another lick of jolly green paint.

To deny the maxim that before defeating prejudice one has to treat the illness virtually borders on the criminal. This is why government policy, excuse the pun, is insane. Twentieth century governments always resorted ultimately to nuclear physics as a learned deterrent to justify the extent to which they could destroy a South Pacific island, but unlike Geoff Hoon, they largely recognized their responsibility to humanity by ending and not initiating a war. In my empty cage of mental health there was similarly a better idea about causes and effects and how dropping a patient from six thousand feet would usually result in an explosion. Even Maggie Thatcher must have grasped that diffusing a bomb first is far more preferable than evacuating seven million head scratchers at dawn from a big city. And so it was that in the 1990s a care in the community approach thwarted the unthinkable properties of untreated mental illness before you were buggered. And with such talent dotted sporadically around the fringes of the jungle, Care in the Community was a realistic hope for those of us who needed expert help.

In 1992, after I had recovered my sanity from the recesses of Hell, and with my mother sitting beside my hospital bed wondering whether this miracle would ever take place, I did not know the formbook. However, although I had turned the corner, I knew and felt that my life was still very far from being salvaged. My trauma after the horror of what had been happening stared back at me straight out of a lion's mouth, and I was severely depressed by it. I couldn't write a logical sentence without any insight or emotions to obey, and it was like I had only managed to scale a prison cell ledge to see a narrow slit of daylight land at my feet. To the Hither Green nurses pacing the corridors, there was no discernable change, and I was still catatonically clinging to the lounge armchair, in fear that if I shuffled one inch, then God would assault me with a kitchen knife. My bewildered family generously came to this exact location at 5pm every day, and Mr. Payton arrived unexpectedly after a five-year absence. However it was rapidly becoming pleasant to converse with an old friend in the leafy grounds, as the adult I had transformed overnight into, and not as the scolded child I had miraculously ceased to be. Andy informed me later that when he referred to Mr. P. about this incident, he had remarked "there is nothing wrong with him, just mega-depressed." Could that be the underlying truth? The medication being pumped into me like an oilfield, was to calm down an normally calm person, and was clearly the source of massive discomfort and an ensuing depressive state. I had been taking Clopixol and Depixol injections for over one year and it felt like I had been asleep for over three quarters of it. The kind of sleep attrition imposed on me by the drugs was not cosy or safe from Dr Zarkov; it was practically a trance-like state of living death, smashing my cheekbones with its angry elbows. The doctors were diagnosing my condition as catatonic schizophrenia, which in layman's terms is a stiffening of a delusional mind, which they had prescribed quite blasphemously. My tongue was not yet loosened enough to point out that their research was pigeon-soup, and if I lost my temper about it, they would gather round, hold a conference and frenetically pin me cheek high to the bed and inject me into Walter Mittyworld. Once upon a time they managed to 'sedate' me for 36 hours, and I am conscious of this because when I woke up early one Friday morning, I still believed it was Wednesday. Some drugs had the opposite effect on the patients by making them restless by encouraging them to goose-step around the hospital like a herd of pigeons all looking for a breadcrumb. These heroes would only have their batteries recharged with further treatment when, through exhaustion they had retired to their cubicle still with the worn out soles to their boots on and their laces tied; for me it was the opposite. My legs felt like ancient Egyptian obelisks, enduring a maddening, muscle stiffness. My feet felt like two icy slabs being whacked by a torturous hammer. I needed a zimmer frame to help me pace up and down. I would imminently leave the hospital bedlam, and without treatment being forced by legislation, my hopes were inaudibly sky-high that my newfound sanity could carry me into a normal life. Three years later I would be crouching on this living room layout like it was an operating table writhing in agony, literally praying to a merciless God that He would take the jabbing pain away from my crippled legs. When I received no feedback I kindly requested for him to take His plaything there and then.

Hither Green was not Manderley and its housekeepers were very far from Danversarian. Nurses came in all shapes, appearances and ages, many of who were female and they gave patients a comfortable ride through magnified desperation. The first to equate with me was everything a person like me might have been, had I been a girl. She was merely twenty-one and possessed the maturity I lacked in the distant three year gap between our ages. My self-esteem casually reminded me that nobody learns from a brush-off with death, only from good thoughts and happy experience personified by this eminently desirable petite blonde from Cardiff who was already claimed. Nobody could have been more proud to have this warm and funny girl for a wife or daughter. On arrival before the miraculous erasure of cracked insanity from my head during the Germany versus Denmark fixture of the 1992 European Championships in Sweden, she showed me constant care and consideration like she was on sentry-duty in Whitehall Palace, which, however prostrate I was, I still didn't think I deserved. Immediately she welcomed me with professional courtesy, which soon snapped under the weight of a sensitive curiosity. This unshaven, unwashed and verbally incommunicado catatonic amazingly intrigued somebody, and I felt grateful that I was vaguely important. I was afforded the usual pleasantries, shown my usual cubicle which consisted of a a three-tier set of wooden drawers, a naff orange plastic chair and a single spring bed, all surrounded by a lovely view of a protective shower curtain. The corridor that divided the twenty cubicles ran about five cricket pitches from the electronically coded security doors to the Victorian washing facilities which still housed two twin baths with steel taps. As a patient continued his pacing up and down he passed three huge window frames whose bars probably eluded his dreamy attentions. The TV room lacked the readymade facilities at Great Yarmouth, but it was pure joy to walk down a patterned red carpet, instead of the slippery wet lino that shone back at the floorwalker with a satanic intensity. Meals were wheeled in on the stroke of 5 o'clock in full view of the office lingering behind the contents of the trolley, whose overlords were busily discussing how to wrap sandwiches in Baco-foil, and still give an injection, while we ate unsupervised.

The patients were usually mild-mannered and unquarellsome. I have made lasting friendships with supposed nutters who like anybody, have simply been down on their luck to give them reason to admit themselves onto a ward to get assistance. Nutters can range from the bereaved to the separated. Hardly nutters don't you think? On my visits to hospital there was almost a code of honour among thieves, whose key strategy was acceptance. Most felt that as soon as they picked up they could return as normally to life as they dared to. The young nurse from Cardiff, Myfanwy, had her wits about her and saw to the sinking ship as soon as I was vaguely coherent. There was no immediate assessment from her as she kindly slugged my few belongings on to my spring bed for me and with a real sense of overwhelming compassion in her eyes she went about her way with objective analysis reflecting truth and faith. All anybody could say candidly was, "I wish I knew what was going on in there" and she pointed to my head as she carefully whispered these sublimely caring words. Without getting carried away, her constant attention could not explain why I broke through the wall of Hell inside me two weeks later, but I do believe that Myfanwy had enough understanding of schizophrenic people to shine a little light and love that no doctor's textbook could supply.

Sandy, the ward sister was a phlegmatically understanding Scottish lady of around thirty, with flowing brown locks and even proportions. She chose her words cautiously, without window-dressing, and spoke in a low vigil that had ensnared patients' trust for many centuries of her working life. Her wily self-experience never super-imposed itself and she got results without being judgmental. My grandmother worked as a ward sister in a psychiatric unit, but she always confirmed that the only difference between the patients and her was the uniform, which I fear, may have been slightly exaggerated, but still, Sandy's disposition felt marvelously symmetrical to traditional modes of NHS care. It soon became obvious to Sandy that my behaviour was becoming socially acceptable quicker than they got through hypodermic assassinations, and she suggested that I might think about moving out to supported accommodation. She had got to know a man called David Walker some years ago when he managed an old people's home next door to her previous address, and now it seemed he ran a mental health unit in Bishopsthorpe Road, Sydenham, not one bus-stop away from where my parents resided and my old school. She was convinced that it was a perfect opportunity to start again for a twenty-four year old, needing full-time care and convalescence. My mother and father who were afraid of my antics at home unsurprisingly threw their wholehearted backing behind the scheme, and encouraged me to shout for the vacancy in the hostel that had recently become available to me. Andy describes my saving grace as being objectivity, and with this resource I understood that they weren't abandoning me like the other poor hospital patients who had been left to fend for themselves alone against stress, and I had no objections to the plan in any case.

The Section 3 of the 1983 Mental Health Act runs for twenty-eight days and for twenty seven of mine, I was rooted to the armchair cushion out of a compulsive, dying wish to keep myself alive. Although a canister lighter in sanity, my trip through God's psychological smog fest still bounced at right angles like a rapier through my soul. Sandy knew I was better because I communicated enthusiastically, and read Myfanwy's tactically probing questions before she could finish the sentence. However my posterior never left the armchair to convince anybody who knew me that I was not altogether of sound mind. When confronted with food I was forced to leave my seat which gave me confidence to return to my bunk for an uninterrupted twelve hour sleep and yet I did not consider rationally that whenever I stood up to disobey His commands, God would surely pursue me to the brink. In the hours of sunny daylight I walked the grounds with Myfanwy's attendance, which I imagined rather inappropriately like chintzing martini glasses with your favourite Hollywood model under the Parisian moonlight. When I invested too close in her beauty however, she became the vacant model of indifference sealing the impassable boundaries between us. I had lovingly compiled a thousand piece jigsaw only to lose the missing piece of the puzzle right at the end of my mission, and I was too fed up by my determined devotion to duty to start the game again. While I could hear the raunchy echo of

Tchaikovsky's Romeo and Juliet from the sand she beat it up and over Beachy Head to avoid my clinched fingers. I must have been uglier than I thought for her to behave like this. I shamefully compared my rejected countenance to 'his' again in mourning. Not Brad Pitt or Hatty, but the lad who had ceased to exist on the Norfolk Terrace stairwell six years before when he needed fly spray to keep the adoring female temptresses at bay. Myfanwy had rejected me but did not know 'him'. She didn't know the truth about who 'he' really was beneath the shabbily dressed, crooked man he had become. How could I show her the truth when all that I could adopt was rejection for what I had spuriously materialized into. Even the memory of that slim, well-proportioned, smiling, attractive younger 'him' had died in abject obscurity. With every pint sunk, curry gorged, and chocolate bar chomped, the superficial anti-hero became a doormat for every rasping 'no' delivered at a romantic, tragic, bloated wreck staining him far more in blood than common. Despite the logical truth evading the misguided perception of my features, I did learn an important truth about ladies in horse racing terms in that they will only back favourites.

Hospital ennui was only marginally pierced by visiting hours which helped me relax my attention towards Myfanwy's whistle while you work while down a coalmine attitude to her daily chores. One evening at about 7 o'clock typically without prearrangement, two agreeable looking strangers dressed like undergraduates, whisked me off to the staff office laced with breadcrumbs that Myfanwy had not resorted to sweeping for the other staff to discuss reconnaissance with a view to accepting the Bishopsthorpe vacancy. I could see they were more honest than image conscious which I have always preferred and it was quite amusing that rather than broadcasting an upbeat frivolity, both looked candidly miserable, as if the world was about to dislodge from their shoulders and disintegrate. One man explained that he was the co-manager of the hostel with Dave Walker and that he had left the Rolls outside, only bothering to dress in faded denim jeans and a grey acrylic cardigan because they were his work clothes. Colin had a round face more in contempt of himself than anybody else, and his John Lennon style spectacles hid nothing of the understanding look in his eyes that suggested the world betrayed one and all. The rest was a solid question and answer interview session that I seemed to prevail in. I fell immediately for the lack of conditions to occupy me at the hostel, despite being distracted by my grim illusions of leaving the armchair to risk my entire sanity and so I tentatively requested to visit the hostel before I made a definite decision, although if God didn't reinstate my madness I would have gone there on the first morning bus out of Hither Green. Simon Williams, the other interviewer who was a crack social worker, and who had been loaning expert recommendations to mental health institutions longer than Hither Green had been a hospital, cheerily ran his fingers through his dense black beard, while Colin inspected his steamed up glasses, wiping and investigating them for the hundredth time, thereby agreeing to my illogical reservations, and invited me to their chambers: It appeared like I was in.

However unless I received a firm push there was no other way I was going to recover from my armchair fixation to make a clear cut decision in my favour. If I had been offered the crown jewels I would have dithered until a schizophrenic signal fooled God into allowing me to swipe them. The storm clouds were gathering behind the latest 200mg injection of Depixol to supposedly liberate me into taking the gamble. Without a stimulus I could not act until all reasonable doubt was taken away, and then when she walked through the secure doors with Colin at heel she gave me one I shall never forget. Six days swept by repeatedly with only Myfanwy, my heart's desire, postponing the weary whitewashed walls that invaded my catatonic stare, and the iron girder bars on the windows from strangling me. Trolleys held a peculiar fascination for world watchers whether they be delivering gourmet lunches from Heinz, confectionery from the dearest of dear old dears, or enough medication to feed a small army. She came, as I was about to have my spuds.

It made a startling limited appeal on my sexually dulled senses to see this stonking set of pegs spin through the world's most padded cell in need of a lift. Initially, I pressed my heart-beating lust defensively into the grey familiarity of the blank walls behind me. I did acknowledge that she looked fabulous however, with beauty and sex emitting from her toenails. My decision was reached when she came close enough for me to see that she was without doubt the horniest woman I had ever seen. She was the type of girl that you wanted to escape a lunatic asylum to be with only for her to put you straight back in institutionalized surroundings six months later. The tail I never knew I had started wagging like a puppy dog and my mouth turned to leather as my tongue automatically disobeyed my brain's commands by gravitating six times round the Sun. In the mad breath of reality, Colin exposed Liz as a Bishopsthorpe client whose presence uprooted the riotous fixation I had developed for a tufty armchair, and for the first time in my life I was free, like I had been living in a box, but only to escape to world that needed handling with care.

I was not jumping from a late Victorian institution to a late Victorian institution either, although I would have worn an iron mask to share any space with Liz. The first stop on day release was the Spotted Cow, a popular rounding up point for absconders down Hither Green Lane during this muggy Summer. Over a couple of light refreshers in the pub garden my lust throbbed deliciously for the picture postcard queen, wearing a revealing, patterned 'thingie' that left little to my dormant imagination. Unless I was blind Bishopsthorpe had to be a more appealing risk by the second. I kept my singular thoughts under my hat as Lizzie delicately handled the stretch limo through the onrush of Catford's one-way bottlenecks and pelican crossing queues, back to our base. She spoke pleasantly but routinely to me like any old newcomer to a family fold while she stubbed the remains of a lighted fag into the ashtray just below the gear lever. I could perhaps impress upon her no more than the mental health survivor I had been officially declared as. Colin drenched these romantic initiatives in a timely, long-winded dialogue about what I could expect as I bowled up an untrodden path to the sturdy yellow front doors, in a local Sydenham street I knew well enough to have had dreams of living in since I was a small kid. Bishopsthorpe Road was part of the esteemed Thorpe Estate whose multi bedroom properties were set to sore in the wave of booming housing markets in the 1990s. The roads were noiseless and clean and despite backing on to a similarly enchanting busy high street, never disorderly. Bishopsthorpe could be as follicular as Primrose Hill or any sleepy village and presently with even the front door giving off the rays of the sun, and the four tiers of respectable late Victorian masonry stretching heroically up for its ecstatic embrace, I had to pinch myself.

The mysterious whereabouts of David Walker was not automatically obvious. Colin and Lizzie ghosted me into the sitting room via the paneled hall floor way, and it was arranged like many typical middle-class homes would be in that district. There were two three-seater loungers, one with a beige, cotton throw over masking its elegance, and one leather armchair almost suffocated by the back door which opened onto an unweeded but not densely overgrown garden. On the yellow walls behind the semi-circle of furniture stood some laughably cheap looking pictures, screaming and begging to be replaced. Below the high white ceiling on the floor lay an expensive dappled rug which leant a beautiful warmth to a room already steaming from the blissful heat bending soothingly through the backdoor's wooden window frames. There was a bookshelf hiding behind a large widescreen TV and in the far corner lay a tasteless coffee table which spread-eagled several small ashtrays for all those who sucked. I saw no radios but the room was clean and it smelt nice. My stare followed Liz down through a small gully as she exited to her own den bolting the door behind her, and I noted a small pantry practically adjacent full of last ditch supplies on its shelves like custard powder and tinned meatballs. Colin sat me down with a rakish looking client, who was tall, well-built and dark. His ungroomed hair bounced off his scalp like it was plugged in. He wore old jeans and scratched, white trainers, and could not have been older than thirty-five. He was following intensely the action from the Barcelona Olympics, which I had been watching with avid fruitlessness on the Churchillian set in the hospital. He was watching, however, a satellite channel, and with his big leg outstretched over the sidearm and resting on the slippery backdoor glass, he had evidently been involved in the all-day coverage since the morning hour. He looked handy and his approach to newcomers rang alarm bells. Without diverting the slightest attention from Chris Boardman's epic rides round the Velodrome, he pasted me with a series of personal interview questions as his left leg slumped down the back door pane of glass. I answered his sheet of formal and personal questions as nerve janglingly and as accurately as I could, after Myfanwy's eighth degree had schooled me in the art of political evasion, and I figured that his prurience had clearly been bought from a similar benefactor in his mental health history. I didn't immediately dislike him but he could forget any overtures of friendship. I reasoned that the other three clients Colin had warned me about would regulate the odds of being struck by this rather course looking intimidator who was vulgarly swigging down his Kronenbourg four pack. We both relaxed our guard when he offered me one of his "tubes" to turn away the July heat and turn my attentions on to the cycling. The intoxicated stranger was not sipping down the Special Brew by the dozen. That was Colin's party. He was perhaps generous and sober enough then, not to be an alcoholic. I enjoyed four cans of the amber fluid before I knew what had hit me and then the light slowly barged its way through the overhanging treetops in Mayow Park immediately behind the garden wall. The crude wally who was to be my imminent guardian and welfare advisor was none other than David Walker. Then as I blinked away the shock, giggling internally at the humorous twist to my stupidity, Colin blithely delved into his trouser pocket to crack open a can of Tennants!

11

I was respectfully introduced to the other two clients mid-afternoon who joined us in the legendary debating chamber for a medication-inflicted snooze. Sahara seemed friendly and looked like she had dug her experienced flat heals confidently into many a care joint during her life, and Donny was pleasantly unobtrusive if a little diffident. They shocked me less than the managers of the hostel and I had soon gotten to grips with them and their 'tubes'. To complete the family set was Trixie the overweight team dog, who had been rescued at an auction in Battersea. There the sleeping and the sleeping dogs did lie; all containing mad extremes, colourful and never, ever dull. There was no overall competition to be the best, rivalries or cliques, although it was obvious from the start that Lizzie and myself would go our own way as Sahara and Donny had already done. However, there was enough under this average suburban utopia to attend to the four differing needs of each contender and push the staff well over the edge of the cliff someday. Even the depressed dog was a contributor.

There were many horror stories circulating about hostels well beyond the penniless borough of Lewisham. I had psyched myself up for theft, drug abuse and violence way ahead of Scottish nurse Sandy's suggestion to move away from safety. She had obviously completed enough homework to recommend me to David because of a fondness for both parties who should click. Elsewhere her patients were not so lucky. In other formally regulated hostels, stories were rife that landlords pocketed housing benefits, social security and disability allowances, relaying a meager pittance back to the clients gasping for cigarettes they couldn't afford. The cash, which was paid to the clients by name, was never reinvested into their living quarters, their clothing or their meals, but by default into privately booming bank accounts and big Mercedes Benz. Within two drinking hours with our feet up watching the telly, I sussed that David and Colin had redistributed more wealth than would last a poor client a week in other grim establishments. Over there, there was no meritorious selection process to correspond to Simon Williams and Colin's interview in Hither Green. Here even the clients were consulted about my reputation and suitability. Over there, when your private fortunes ran out, temporary accommodation was forfeited without mercy while you dodged the broken beer bottles and drug needles deposited by street gangs with unwelcome access to vulnerable people, on your way out. From Catford to Honor Oak and from Forest Hill to Brockley the hoodwinked council did their utmost to line the pockets of malicious and spineless racketeers who wore the badges of ruthless Dickensian moneylenders.

With the most severe of depressions and trauma sinking down below my void mind, body and spirit, and vulnerable to violent threats and intimidation, I could not have coped over there, and would probably have next been admitted to a morgue than Alexandra Ward in Hither Green. However over here in the oxygenized revitalization of Bishopsthorpe Road, I still had no earthly clue of how and when I could get out of the royal chasm. My pain and suffering over Junie was acute and my mind still confirmed the awful unrealities of past schizophrenic psychoses as realities. The doctors diagnosed that I had no insight into what schizophrenia really meant and I was unsure after the Denmark/Germany game whether I still had it. I had no more education how to survive with it now, than I did to soldier on without it. I had lost so much life under the all-enveloping illness and all my dreams had dried up in the sick valley of my death. I could not determine whether my living death was organically imposed by the clotting medication or by an insidious illness, but I felt as lost and afraid as Jonah inside his whale. Perhaps worst of all was that my creative senses had shut down like a disused garage and couldn't rescue my ego. David remarked that I was "mega-intelligent", but for me it felt like I had outlived the moribund writing talent I should have staged when at my peak. My vast intellect should be speaking foreign languages fluently or bringing equanimity from inside the minds of the gluttonous oil barons, and not popping out sporting facts I had memorized on trivia machines. These standards I pushed into Dave's face laid well below the average needed to issue self-respect, and the arguments I presented to his pepped up mind were at most belligerent and failed half truths. In my obnoxious self-denial these wound me up even more even though Colin and David tried to endorse me by not effacing them. Thus I told myself I was a deep loser in pain and afraid I would never get better and stimulate a cloth eared world needing my humour and talents, which lay, chopped under the floorboards of Hell.

By evensong Chris Boardman had won his gold medal, and David relinquished his front row ticket to enjoy another feast in the cramped kitchen area, after he invited me to try his swordfish. I saw no reason to quarrel with a former chef whose victuals were a vital supplement to the gunge Colin said I had been throwing down my neck in Hither Green. For Colin this was as close as it came to laying down the law and as he took a hefty swig of lager I ascertained that if David was the action man, then he was the cutesy teddy bear. In a team that worked Colin did the thinking, and David did the speaking.

When I returned to the hospital three hours later than scheduled, Sandy was on hand to ask dryly if the operation had been successful. I could only grin, half dribbling my intake slowly down the side of my mouth to remind her that swordfish is a lot more satisfying than the medication run I had missed at 9pm. I protested my alcoholic innocence on my breath and remonstrated that I was drooling because of the house, David, Colin and Lizzie and Desmond Lynam. Would anyone like to dance with me? Sandy winked at Zebedee and said it was time for bed. However, first to assuage Him, I sweatily made it over to the sitting room chair to feverishly offer my guilty devotions in return for His lame forgiveness. One or two of the patients spotted around the TV had overridden tiresome female authority to watch some sport. It was highlights of all the Olympic sports events I had seen for free, with the number one sexiest female ever pincering in and out of eyeshot like a magician's assistant, while eating a gourmet dinner with free booze. At the end of the day I felt like Chris Boardman with a gold medal dangling round my neck.

The hospital hours ground me down like the monotonous clicking of a windmill sail, and although my bags were packed, the Ethelred Room, my room, was a world of wood shavings, torn up floorboards and a loo, whose chain flushed upwards. Bishopsthorpe ran with the efficacy of the Trumpton Fire Station, but with the lunacy of a Murray Walker commentary. I was let off the leash a few weeks after my short adventure to the Brickyard, as the discharge papers were sealed setting me free. Whatever the fictional misgivings were of leaving behind my armchair, there was no point hanging on there and turning into a stalactite, particularly as I was cogent enough to twig that Myfanwy was nursing me, and not going to succumb to my feckless adult fantasies. Not even the BBC's shy and retiring tennis correspondent, Terry Wogan, could keep me mentally healthy until the Wimbledon rain abated, despite serving more aces than a Pete Sampras one stroke rally. When it was time to go it felt like the ordeal of a first day at school had ended. The rapport with all the staff had ascended to a mutual appreciation, but I shall always palpitate in horror at the 'other' person who was sitting on his bed in the eye of the storm, before she put it to me that she "wished I knew what was going on in there."

Liz whisked me off with my bin liner of whiffy belongings in David's family saloon, crimson Renault. She was an advanced driver and could negotiate road works like she was riding a bike, despite being rubber-stamped with the dubious honour as a Bishopsthorpe inmate. Dave cared for all persons of negligible status, and was constantly slamming me with the sheen of Tony Payton's cricket bat, that to forge ahead one had to trust, and so he provided incentives for his clients to trust him, by loaning them responsibilities such as the borrowing of his car. David and Colin fed me their ultimatum to "take responsibility" for myself so that I could "self-determine" in the future, when I could enlist in harder activities, the pressure of which would land me flat on my face if not ready. However, stupid is as stupid does, and there was no stipulated time to rush me headlong into tasks I would fail in, so Colin and Dave offered me their unsubdued life-experience as a refresher. Could I trust them? What would be the point of not believing their over-enthusiastic, rough and ready lectures and encouragement? At least I was able to attribute heroic status to them for clearly being on my side when I needed help.

While all the other hostels in Lewisham were run by Arab terrorists, 17 Bishopsthorpe hostel should read 17 Bishopsthorpe hotel. From the outside it was nothing, as somber as Trixie, just a few white window frames beeping like the amber flashlight front door, and a cracked patio in disrepair. I was pleased that my den faced out onto the neighbourly street, so that I wouldn't have to stumble past snoring pets after staggering in from a late night out with Andy. My bedroom was also in spitting distance of the main kitchen, which was officially shut after the hours of 10pm to obey fire regulations, and to deter the hooded late night snacker from raiding the abundantly filled fridge freezer. If in need of a bite during the night each unit did have a miniature kitchenette with coffee making facilities, except that mine was a mountainful of Colin's old Guardians, and impassable after a quiz night out with Andy. With David cooking a la carte, the Baby-Belling stove only applied to Santa in this grotto, if he opened the crimpled newspapers to read Jamie Oliver's section.

My bedroom was also the largest on the four floors and David kindly offered the choice of a double bed, which I declined after a little manipulation away from the impressionable hope that I could hook Liz one night. The three arched windows that processed the sunshine were shrouded by three heavy drapes that could have dangled from a Norman abbey, and each were drawn irreverently by a bell-pull for sumptuous effect. Liz regularly cleaned up my mess who worked freelance at fifty pounds an hour for David, unless world interest rates affected share prices in his pockets, but she came cheaper than Carol Smilie did and without the teeth. David was a cognitive thinker who seemed to read minds like he could cook, and realized he had to assert such ways and means for Lizzie and I to eventually assert ourselves. David was roguish in entirety and according to my mother who was a match for any cognitive saint or sinner, he was always "a strange mixture". However he was a peerless financial expert, who could have procured funds for our welfare, and the continued upkeep of an unbouyant hostel by fishing in the Sudan. When Lizzie developed a soft spot form in her harder shell, and provided a truly sympathetic nature with which to hear my plight, she boldly confided to me "Dave has always been obsessed by money." If this is absolutely true then it made him more of a lifesaver than a sinner. The Bible accuses us again of being evil if we love money, but whoever said that wasn't shopping at the right places! If David had been governor of the Bank of England, his handling of money would have brought more peace and prosperity, and what is wrong anyway than possessing no greater love than laying down his wallet for the sake of his friends?

One of his first exactions was to settle the benefit supports that I should have collected for six straight years of unrelenting illness, and which should certainly have been my right one year after leaving Great Yarmouth hospital without any follow-up care. I had been too proud to collect guilt money, but now it was decided that I really should be compensated to the hilt after my slog around London's dutiful trivia circuit. There was no greater indicator of his genius when he scribbled down on the income support forms that I "had difficulty rotating soiled clothes", and no more deserved inheritor than myself.

Some income was efficiently diverted back into the cost-effective heart of the hotel service. David and Colin collected the monthly cheques and equitable housing benefit, and siphoned off residue for maintenance costs, all bills, the Satellite TV service drafted into everybody's bedroom with full consent, and food and beer consumption. With these outgoings I was still better off because the handsome wedge of pocket money left over, was more than adequate to spend on liberty, without being distracted by the stresses of everyday disasters and mental illness. I couldn't care if the two proprietors made a little on the side here and there, because they worked twenty-four hour shifts, cooking, cleaning, repairing, and arguing with the dogmatic Council to recognize their status, seven days a week. Colin's sagging shoulders at the interview resulted from all the unheralded hours he thought he could have wasted in a normal vocation. He was however a vital influence to the partnership, because his excellent reasoning, could order one of Dave's ideas before it had jumped ship. Colin was also an unsung gofer, who quietly did the chores and kept the debt collectors up the high street happy with a silver tongue, while Dave sorted out the latest cash-flow crisis. Colin was caring and attached to the patients enough for Liz to call him the "mother figure", despite his competence in masculine odd-jobs, and his back pocket full of readies tied together by Jim Bowen, for food-runs, and emergency tooth-aches. Otherwise the duties were evenly shared between the two Mr. Fixits who could instantly turn water into wine if you asked them nicely. Instead of waiting for the TV man to appear in glorious Technicolor, they could chill out in front of the soaps to watch a set they might have tinkered successfully with in the afternoon haste, and deservedly sink a bottle bank of tubes. I was fooled by my overblown first impressions because their behaviour was no more than a reaction to non-stop graft by two very ordinary gentlemen.

The two gladiators (David being Goliath) were no strangers to the devil's advocate, and with Colin sometimes throwing his rustic spanner into the works, capable of some very funny arguments that would have raised awareness in the Houses of Parliament. At this juncture in my personal development I was no match for either's intellectual jousting, but I felt confident enough to interpose when the beer started talking. In the afternoons, Donny, Sahara, and myself as Sodom faced Gomorrah facing each other like the black and white pieces at the start of a chess game, routinely sat through Fifteen-to-One and

Countdown. Dave with his big left boot trailing down the glass panel as usual would offer an insensitive word about Carol Vorderman's sexy legs, before Colin would announce to his public audience that he had 'a six'. At two o'clock in the morning I could just make out through thin walls David questioning the rules and Colin confirming his 'six' in the flaky English dictionary on the bookshelf. What they must have been like at school is anybody's guess. Then first thing in the morning, David would be articulately rambling down the phone at a civil servant and Colin would be proudly hoovering the carpets with a solid mothering. This was just the way it was at Bishopsthorpe.

Although not mad, I was suffering pain's energy, whose yearned release was forfeit, due to a bolted mind interior. I craved crying so badly just to unload the cloying misery of all past experience, but gates of industrial steel barred the dam. There was no psychological release incurred by the agony of no emotional release, like I was the water swirling around an already blocked sink. When the taps of love turned on the sink simply became even more clogged and in danger of erupting. However the love I sought was simply lost, and thoughts simply reinforced the telling failure of my intelligent thought patterns. I staunchly hated the way I was, disregarding the love of my empathic ear, touching the other household members. Without a particular gift I had nothing to promote myself and felt universally unpopular. Since the bleak midwinter of UEA, my self-esteem had risen to −272 degrees.

However, with the chilling sandstorm of madness forever effaced, and allied to the willpower and determination I had counted on in the cesspit, I saw reasons not to hide away anymore. I had a swimming intent to explain my heartless and cruel withdrawal from Junie, and to write to her for rosy forgiveness, before I could start to forgive myself. I could not let my obesity or lack of wit take her by surprise if I met her, so I should write to her with trust and honesty, pre-empting the dismantling of the preconceived hero she idolized. There could be no future to an honest relationship without being immediately up-front. To communicate by letter had always been our flag post, and her disappointment in its softened and unmelodic literary presence could be assuaged, for a resurgence of delight in knowing my whereabouts after six barren years. She would also have no reason to doubt the Milky Bar stuffing 16 stone cake fiend for the cat walking, waif-like teenager she could still imagine. However the need to contact her living spirit was clinched by the agonized passing of time while I had waited to lay my head once more next to the daughter of my hope and strength when the war had raged at UEA. I had no more time to play with because each family-sized Milky Bar I gulched, the quicker the belly flopped out. I consulted a disquieted Dave, who knew his way around women, announcing my strategy before his life-experienced reasoning could shine light on the proposal. I slumped over my high, grey writing desk, with a stack of paper and seven, pristine ballpoint pens for many days, recounting vividly all the schizophrenic horror in detail, shamelessly wafting through the skeletons that hung there in the wind. David offered to correct the intricate stories, which I foolishly attributed to corrupt nosiness, but these had to be my own sorry words, however vulgar. Within a very long weekend, and a bin full of discarded sweet wrappers, my first and only 40 page epic was complete. Junie would never hang a gold medal over my shoulders for the audacious way I had described the person still miraculously known as Rob Morrison, but it gave her a precious choice to embrace him as he is or remember him as he was, and for this reason I thought it was a fair exercise.

The trouble with the contents I had submitted to her old address was that I could not be swayed in my misinterpreted understanding of reality that had passed. I could not be persuaded that God had never intended me to shoot the Queen Mother with a rifle I could not buy or aim straight with. In my schizophrenic Hell, His flagrant orders could not be associated or attributed towards my illness because, through shame, they offered me an escape. God had simply turned up a tempest to an Armageddon. Although entirely justified by previous rationalizations made under the weight of the Terror, God doesn't fit into a non-delusional and normal world of undefined paranoia. In my darkest hours He had revealed no inner light to teach me how to trust Him. The evidence pointed too surely to Great Yarmouth exorcisms and orange juice. Therefore, the only information I was giving June was that I had become my worst history and not escaped from it. I was trapped in the barbed wire netting of the past there to be gunned down in the present. Simon Williams gently supported that she might believe I was crazy, even though my remit for the letter was to indicate that now I was not.

Junie did write a substantial note of three lines back, handwritten on a scrap of A4 lined paper for my amusement, without a trace of sentimentality and loaded with deafening intent. Realistically it was all I expected. The Truth had rejected me, and Dave knew it. Logic told me she had plumped for the soft option from the two choices. She knew her old friend Rob, but not this wicked foreigner who had quite quickly saddened her. I figured it was safer for me that she had torn out the address page from her diary, before the relationship could dwindle away in the flesh, for I too needed to freeze past memories. However the frailty of women assured me that if I drove a Mercedes and had a pop career, she would have been less fickle and more loyal. From that day I was rejected by womankind, probably for an image or danger, and I doubt if she will ever be with a real man again.

However, life without Junie went on even if it was excruciatingly mean not to pay the dividend on my years of dutiful investment. Lizzie could turn my head in primitive backwaters that had yet to sink me. I told myself as she casually flicked her hair and tugged sharply on the gear stick of David's car that she was not deliberately trying to bewitch me. However she was a dirty concoction of three-minute orgasm, and Parade magazine. Lizzie could lasso any steer in a Stetson, but how she could always end up with a mad, gun-slinging outlaw was a calamity. I was simply one of the drunken posse rounded up to wolf-whistle and howl while she danced out of touching distance. Somehow I thought I was different, until I noticed other competitors begging and pleading for her favours in exactly the same way. However, Lizzie and I did pay each other genuine attention and respective compliments which arrowed through the drawbridges en route to our hearts. She liked me and cared about me "more than I could ever know", and she was right. Although I could never perceive it inwardly, it took an outsider to acclaim me as "a genuine bloke". Lizzie taught me that the world saw me in a totally different light to how I saw myself, and I was encouraged to listen more attentively to the warm light shone by those I could trust. This was the point of no return where I actually found a true mate who knew me. Andy and Simon's unfailing loyalty had carried me through the extremes of Hell thus far, but they had homes of their own to build, and I needed new blood to depend on. Lizzie was the beginning, possibly because she was right for me. I was 24.

However, drooling over Liz's skin-tight jogging bottoms blurred the sensible boundaries of observational content. It was made worse by the Depixol injections inhibiting any sexual energy and interplay. Instead of humorising my throbbing lust with a delicate brush, I became contained by unreleasable desires, and came across quite seedily. It seemed like I was thinking what I wasn't thinking. Sex was at my core but became like a dampened sideshow, for which I compensated seduction with overloaded romantic commitment. This was like how I knew what it was to love June without the remotest emotional evidence since my illness. Liz knew I fancied her, but medication had dealt me cards that only a bluffer could deliver. It just wasn't fair.

What gave me a mountain to climb was that I had the renowned 'Community Psychiatric Nurse (CPN) From Hell' to completely ride roughshod over the wailed bleating of all those she inflicted impotence on by injection. It was this lady's job to administer the dose of medication each robotic psychiatrist had cold-heartedly, but wholeheartedly prescribed. There is one reliable story that she was so obsessed with forced treatment that she followed a friend of mine into his local Catford pub, to ask him to drop his trousers before his disbelieving mates had time to sweep up the broken glass. She even opened her briefcase to reveal her magic array of clinical hypodermics, embarrassing my friend's reputation and her own antiquated beliefs by about two hundred years. There was simply no escape and absolutely every reason on earth to avoid confiding in her before it was too late.

12

In the hostel, Sahara and I regularly watched MTV because it compensated for no stereo unit. One afternoon while Sahara was doing her Whitney Houston impressions on the sofa, there was a patronizing knock at the front door, answered by Colin. It was Hecate Hatecrime, come to turn me into a frog. I was delirious. She was shown in to the sitting room where I was struggling to hold a mug of hot tea, with stage fright. My back remained turned to the angel of horror behind me as I mimed along to a Def Leppard song which was featuring on the satellite music channel. Hatecrime sweetly misinterpreted the whole straightforwardness of normal behaviour, by announcing within earshot to Colin, that "he's talking to himself again". I never talked to myself, even when my time of one second was up, and she fetched out a hypodermic the size of Cleopatra's Needle, for me to worry about. In view of my sexual needs, this was like giving glucose to a diabetic. Injections moreover, clatter the nervous and sexual systems for over a month, so it was obvious that if I let this mad bitch off her chain, I would squander any realistic hope of bagging Lizzie for further painful weeks. The composite answer within mental health teams to "I'm impotent", is, "You're depressed", but I can honestly suggest without referring the case to the Idiot's Complaints Committee (for racial equality), that I was depressed because I was impotent and not impotent because I was depressed. Fact has lain unresearched by every last one of my support workers because they have been too blind and not caring enough to dispute the truth. Every time I cry that medication is not infallible, I am greeted by the shuddering echo of "But..." it's not that they are not open-minded enough to believe me, it's just that they never will. Too risky.

Invisibly and surreptitiously, Liz was weaving a magic spell on yet another piece of toast, and I had to confront Dave about my limited sexual appetite before she became too familiar and left me for unleavened bread. I had to relax the medication to stiffen my resolve. Depixol gave me absolutely zero quality of life in all respects ("But...!"). My eyes were so tired that they almost dropped off, screening a view of reality's light from the pitch-black darkness of an underground mining tunnel. I slept through more day-to-day existence than Ronald Reagan, and I shook like a workman's pneumatic drill, which is kindly, jargonized as 'involuntary spasms.' I could never settle or concentrate while my legs manically peddled around the moon exhaustively. Furthermore my hands trembled violently and my mouth jutted around like stretched elastic. This was noted in the professional handbook as being a 'Parkinsonian' defect brought about by anxiety. The health manuals advised a patient to consult a doctor if suffering from the side effect of nervous ticks, but whenever I consulted a doctor, he never consulted the health manuals. But.. It got so out of hand when I had escaped Hatecrime's claws that I had to waste NHS time by seeking counselors with psychological fractures that had been caused by the NHS. Then all they would prescribe was a further course of medication. Liz was never going to be single for more than five minutes, and the depression my defeat caused would leave further room for more treatment in the future costing money and resources. David at least backed down, and agreed to the dangerous diversion of a paranoid schizophrenic abating his medication.

Private counselling sessions were arranged by the hostel because there was no facility in the Lewisham and Guy's Mental Health Trust, which is odd considering the overwhelming demand, but unfortunately commonplace. Until then the solitary ear was the psychiatrist, whose only job description I soon found, was to tranquilise and deaden down any inherent ability with rhetoric about the usefulness of drugs having 'rave reviews.' I feared going to doctors who wouldn't last five minutes on their own prescriptions, because if I told the truth, they would either send me down to Hither Green or make me even more impotent. Since I didn't want either and usually got both, the private counsellor was an alternative that was literally forced upon me.

It was the first time I had communicated my troubles since I had started university, before which I had nonesuch troubles to communicate. I had six sessions before pulling out. The counsellor was good but my wounds too grievous, and my entrails too spilled. Catford was always grim but safer than today, and after rocking my foundations I would wander through its backstreets towards home in a daze with my scrambled head pointing the wrong way, and my mind caving in on itself. One night after I had caught the 202 bus back to Sydenham, I had to plead with Colin to calm me down again in the Golden Lion, to alleviate the multitude of stress that had cropped up in the counselling session. Colin downed tools at ten o'clock to do this much against his will, but out of kindness and to prevent any nonsense becoming, affrayed nonsense.

Stumbling around the Thorpe Estate, frequently afforded time for positive reflection and I became aware of the narrow and steep pathway down from my dizzy traumatisation. Where the path began and how I lasted its course was the problem. Life was stable but not becoming easier, but that is why I needed care. Thankfully Bishopsthorpe care was not imposed like all the other hostels in the region. If I could only stagger from my bed like a cadaverous shell at the crack of midday, then it was forgivable, and likewise if I trashed my room with sweet papers and soiled clothes. To society's anxious ears I was lazy, but my professional housemates could discern my determination to procure a future as soon as I could step out of this messy present. However this moment could never let go of its past, so I was unable to fulfill my task in this way. The present was too horrifying to commit to, because it regressed to Junie, like I was skating on the brink of jagged ice.

It was decided that after seven months of yawning renouncement of immediate hope that I could be allowed to experiment with my medication intake for an interluding period. It was satisfying just to get one over on Hecate whose attitude to the whole world being on Depixol was unemployed. I had administered anti-psychotic medication for two years without the respite of a normal life. Under its influence, your thought processes were so scotched that you couldn't differentiate between what was real and what wasn't. Doubt about who you were and what you were, multiplied faster than Hecate's advice could reinforce it. I had no more knowledge of who I was than what my body was doing 'involuntarily', to disobey my disintegrating mind. Medication was no life and I prayed that my sanity would be more effective against mental illness than my bleeding system

However my resources to fill the vacant corridor of uncertainty were not replete enough to withstand it. Hecate's pressurising obsession didn't help by ordering me by post on a daily basis to proceed to her office and receive two hundred jabs for passing no-go. I lost the fight because I submitted to obsessional behaviour that I could have resisted. If I had not undone myself, I could have had long-intended sex, a slicker waistband, and all the creative flair I needed, but God implacably rubbed it in my face once again. Without medication He unjammed the hotline and reinstituted the idea of shaming myself to beat my illness. At first He confused the ambitious impression I had made on Liz, as yet unblemished and without darkness. I was dying inside without her, but was still savvy enough not to overreach the desired outcome by tossing myself into the abyss. It was cruel enough already without taking her with me, but God did enough to damage and humiliate my reputation in her eyes alone to be perfectly glorious.

He sustained the idea in me that Liz would one day have my children. It was a pleasurable thought without a shred of evidence, which normally a mild schizophrenic would discard as nonsense. I was no different, but God condemned right-minded freewill, by convincing me I had to tell her. This was a tragic leap, for when I anxiously did tell her, Liz became quite petrified of the friend she thought she knew, but didn't. We became strangers overnight, and I became depressed, stressed and overtly intent on redressing the wound. Without medication, the irony was I could still keep well enough to obey the laws of freewill, but if somebody predicted or promised a desired outcome with Liz, I would overturn any objective inhibitions to achieve it. Since God now controlled my mind's destiny He was free to embarrass me in any destructive way He decreed.

To gain Lizzie, God commanded that I stay in bed all day, scream the 'Neighbours' theme tune, hop around on one leg and pee up the wall or face rejection. I could have behaved as sanely and sensibly as before, but the stakes offset the merciful freedom of mind, body and spirit, that detoxication would allow. My brain was not yet addicted and with David and Colin's supervision, I could have recovered full composure, before it was too late to proceed with a normal life. The cost of obeying God and not my sanity it hardly needs saying was prolific, and probably culminated in a foreshortened life.

After two more bedridden weeks, I lay stagnant in stinking clothes before God insisted I yelp for help at my highest pitch. It was still in my power to dress and wash myself and sustain normal conversation with the other housemates, but God had gripped my mind like a yellow fever and there was no way out. Colin and David unlocked my bolted door and were speedily to the rescue. Social Services were notified not a second later. However this was late Friday afternoon, and the proprietor's task was handicapped by emergency staff only rigidly available during office hours. Therefore I had to be restrained until Monday morning before I shot off down the high street in just a pair of black jeans to sit provocatively in a burger bar. I pushed past them eagerly before the long arm of David's law made an arrest. Naturally enough, apart from being a trained chef and a general handyman, he had served in the flying squad, and it was not smart to put up resistance. God offered me one final chance to rescue my children when He told me to go berserk, but I had just enough faltering gumption to realize that David would be more likely to expel me than wallop me back, and that was even less alluring. If I had lost my tenancy now, I would have been a martyr to the suicidal consequences of living in the registered hostels in Lewisham. That I disobeyed the Holy Father was a telling twist against Fate defining my life. There was talk of putting me in the nick overnight for my own safety, but somehow I calmed myself down and rested till Saturday morning when Dave ferried me down to the shores of Hither Green in the Renault's royal procession.

Alighting from the car proved a backbreaking ordeal for the six feet two inch copper, without any nurse offering their services to him. Under the 1983 Mental Health Act, a patient could admit himself on to the ward voluntarily if there was clearance and sufficient bed space. Dave gesticulated his carrot aloft, promising fairly that if I took an injection now, I could "still be out in a couple of days." Not following his advice would entail another twenty-eight day section, which would ground me by law, no matter how speedy the recovery. However God insisted that should I observe this sound policy, He would murder my unborn children, so I ended Dave's last-gasp but futile operations and stupidly got readmitted to Alexandra Ward.

Returning to the medical fold was like a welcome home, even if Myfanwy had jumped ship to marry her lover in Pakistan. The familiar old nurses were disappointed to see me back, but compared with the last time, it felt like a holiday camp, especially as I was sectioned under the false pretences of God's holy orders. I knew now how to be cared for, and what it felt like to push the right buttons for room service. I cast my mind back to the shadows of Great Yarmouth where all the patients seemed so optimistic. I was now able to cope satisfactorily like they did, and communicate to our cellmates warmly about what I would do when I got out. It was purely my sanity which enabled me to put into perspective this less than desirable pickle.

I was still however, petrified of medication which would ground me for every month I was injected. To avoid this pitfall, my beliefs had to distort to cling on to God's get-out-clause of salvation. My schizophrenia was entering a psychotic phase free from pain, which I had not grown accustomed to. Consequently when I was ill the front of my cursed and jumbled mind superseded the ordered logic of self-control in my ordinary consciousness. God was always the trigger to destabilize because I had read that His divine purpose was unfailing for me, and could be explained in its greater wisdom which had incited my peculiar behaviour.

The duty psychiatrist was another elegant Persian whose

mind was scientific rather than humanistic, and he flattered his flock with diagnoses between 10 and 12 on Tuesday mornings and not while he was playing golf, during which time our communication skills had rotted under the spate of forcible treatment. His elegance seemed to inspire a brigade of teenage girl students who seemed to swing by the threads of his tweed jacket buttonholes like he was David Essex, and not like the conveyor belt of predictions that earned him sixty grand per year. After further experimentation on me with injections, he warmly advised me that I didn't know how seriously ill I was, which was an attack he made on all patients encouraging them to feel useless. Dr Sess sermonized that I couldn't even imagine the scale of my mountain peak still unconquered, but I wondered where he expected me to be since my invalid university education. It was only clear to me as his diagnosis swept past my ears, that he had never teetered on the brink of a chasm, fallen, and then mountaineered straight back up again. When had he ever taken Clopixol? Dr Sess did not know that day that he had been talking to a survivor, not a loser.

Sess had been headhunted by Janssen Pharmaceuticals who had developed a new drug in tablet form called Risperidone, which strangely enough had been acquiring some 'rave reviews.' After completing scientific research on its guinea pigs, he ended up prescribing it to the entire psychiatric squad in Lewisham. Sess said he would be willing to discharge me from hospital on the one condition that I underwent the tests for this as yet unconfirmed medication. It was corrupt blackmail but an option I was only too willing to take, particularly as he argued there was "no side-effects." I signed my life away to the programme immediately to escape the mind-tyranny Dave had wisely warned me about, and returned to the safe haven of the hostel.

My relationship with Lizzie was already strained by my wobbly conduct, and her aversion to what she had seen, made her skeptical towards me. The castle ruins could never be reconstructed, and I felt as, jaded, confused, deflated and innocent as when my old school friend Paulie had died in a road accident. Her history had feted some of the most barbaric suitors in Christendom, and now she veered her attentions away from this careful and kind weirdo, into the shop-window along Railton Road. It was painful for myself in the short-term and her in the long run that she ceded to the inevitability of more violence, before I could save her. I wept metaphorical tears in frustration, which negative self-esteem surrendered as the damning come-uppance of being a nice guy. Liz, however was the most intelligible of the clientele and had to outgrow Colin and Dave more quickly before shattering into sad, old ways. I surmised that the writing was on the wall when her "so nice" new boyfriend took her to see a low-budget prequel to the Texas Chainsaw Massacre on their first date. Lizzie was strangely always the last one to know when life awarded her its victim's manual for the year. She freely admitted that it was no good if anybody or I never laid a glove on her because she was "addicted" to the danger of violent men. The excuse was more than I could understand from a God who had painted the Mona Lisa and then smeared it with funny glasses and a false moustache. My Liz was leaving the good and placid home to seek her fortune in the dim and gloomy cells of the Bastille and I would miss her.

The Risperidone tablets were a tough drug to force down, like heroin is tricky to kick, but the colony of side effects did not endanger my life completely, and always were just manageable. Simply, the same side effects applied, but their severity was halved. I had got to trust Colin and David quite well through the crisis, when they had visited me everyday with clean washing and formed escape committees to the Spotted Cow with the audacity of Steve McQueen. They insisted firmly that it was not in my interest to bet against the wheel, but to stomach the diet of new tablets, now that I was able to. My intellectual strength could survive the hapless demands of my persecuted body to resist medication, and my objectivity could always be relied upon to weigh up the consequences. Once again, according to Andy it was my "saving grace". Because the hostel owners were not legally supposed to supply medication themselves, I was required to take responsibility for my mental health, by administering the treatment under my own auspices, which ultimately resulted in more freedom to experiment with doses and being educated by any mistakes thereof.

The accommodation-related needs of each client were maintained manfully. I could talk to each proprietor about golf and silly things under the shelter of a more serious environment for important things, like getting well. They were inordinately experienced in life, like two great Buddha's whose words of wisdom instructed a new recruit to the rules of the temple. I could admit that I only had to learn from them to be on their wavelengths one fine day, so I profiled their non-conformist, intellectual lectures like I was back at school. David listed me down a little enviously and somewhat amazingly as 'Goldenballs' because I had taken my madness out on the golf ball he had solemnly seen parring the championship course at Addington, and because I was "good looking". He was the loveable rogue with six series of Lovejoy behind him, surely? The Goldenballs tag felt ridiculous and uncomfortable as a failure, but perhaps a little later as a success, the same tag would sit more proudly. I have learnt that interpreting the hazards of life as an optimist is far more favourable than being a pessimist; it's just much harder to do. Patience is key.

In the downstairs lobby intervening between the kitchen and my bedroom fire door, leant a tall, elongated mirror to a cut a dash in if you were optimistic Dave, or be an object of loathing if you were pessimistic like me. When I shrank past its shimmering radiance it seemed to haul me in backwards like a fishing rod seizing on my curiosity. Liz never deigned to look at it twice as she bounced onwards with tidy corkscrew perm, pert tits and firm waistline. For my ego, the humiliation resembled the climax to the Marathon Man movie where the Nazi is forced to munch his own diamonds by a Jew. Olivier gave up 'svallowing' but I had to endure hundreds and thousands of the little beggars. Whatever David's subtle lies and gentle encouragement, they would be betrayed by the stark reality in the mirror every morning, afternoon and evening. My bloated cheek lines confessed to the Milky Bar addiction, my eyes squinted from the darkness of my soul, and my T-shirt so bumpy from the jelly inside, rode up to my navel above, releasing a two inch gap of hairy flesh for Lizzie to lick her lips at. Sahara compared me to pop sensations Take That, but rather cruelly inferred I was the Gary Barlow clone among his four girl-grabbing backing dancers. In other words I was the misfit, and that fitted conveniently into my mode of thinking. David was wrong for once, and for once Sahara had to be right.

To David and Colin I also lived up to the mysterious tag of 'Goldenballs' on the sports park. I had forgotten completely how to improvise over the chessboard and played like a beginner, learning step by step from a book. However David judged that I could still "play from memory." I had resigned from competitive chess because I could only function from memory which was not sufficient to perform with or enjoy the game with, alone. While my thought processes were uncreative and uninspiring, I had simply transformed into a plodder going through the motions. Colin was of no fewer standards than me, but due to my overt reputation, he had talked himself out of a winning gambit before he had pushed his first pawn. If only tournaments were like that. Our games were as tight and symmetrical as they were sparkless and soulless, but I knew he was about to crack first and blunder, when he would immortally utter in blind panic and confusion, that "I'm losing this!' Yet still in spite of my mediocrity I was affixed with 'Goldenballs'!

I played one last cricket season with mixed results. I was a pale shadow of what had preceded, but I was still pitched into the Marlborough first team more out of hope than destiny. The entire club accredited any batsmen playing wild wahoos over midwicket with the terminology that "his head has gone". Whether or not this applied to my slow psychiatric progress I was not sure, but I laughed and used the term myself all the same. However, my old buddies never stuck the knife in personally and made positive allowances for my reckless play, even lowering the cost of my match fee to accord with my more modest circumstances. The heart never leaves that little village club in Dulwich Common, with its hazy views of sundown overlooking the circular surroundings of wild gorse, its pavilion, and its camaraderie of patterned deckchairs and clink of iced lager glasses. It replicated the unique atmosphere of Lord's and it was a similar privilege to pad up and walk out to bat there, whether the head had gone or not.

If it hadn't been me, I would have laughed at the beer-bellied oaf who couldn't run because of the leg stiffness enforced by Risperidone, but my friends lips swore only to rein in the stray sheep from the herd to protect me from predators and to maintain the sense of whole. Rather than run a mile from the schizophrenic shell some had grown up with, my teammates still respected me above all else as a cricketer.

Some were even kind enough to give away kit. The captain's gamble started to pay dividends and rather than an individual legend, I became a valued spare part to the team. However, I never performed quite well enough either for mine or David's satisfaction, who secretly had advanced extra tea and beer expenses. Dave's tips about not giving my wicket away after getting a good start were parental, but always of good heart, although it was clear his analysis of my batting technique was as flawed as my wild slogs. The unstoppable truth was that I was still too heavy and my miserable legs too crablike, for me to enjoy playing. Rather than therapeutic, it was still depressing to be a part of the old 'him' who brought the folks out of the bar as he followed the confident lessons of his batting master, Viv Richards. 'His' ability should have peaked in 'his' mid twenties. I was disillusioned by the game I couldn't play, so I quit before I ceased to care about or love it as a supporter. It was a wicket/maiden to my mental illness. However in time I have reflected fortunately about the courage and stubbornness that didn't fail me through the inconsistency and lethargy that unjustly ended my premature career. They were characteristics any batsman including Sir Viv, would have sold his soul for, if he had been fit. As I raise a glass of Belgian ale, I shudder with pride that I combated personal darkness as one of my generous peers, and shared my cricketing prowess on the sports field neither as an outsider or a bystander at any time. I had simply traded the 'old man's' talent for endeavour and determination needed to build a better person. This was the real me, and I know this person as contentedly as any 17 year old prodigy or university wicket keeper.

I needed help. I was starving from above and below my forty-inch waistline, brought about by the medication's limitations. I needed to release all the dried tears of the emotional junkyard. I was only exhibiting outward indifference amid a cutthroat and bloodthirsty hunger to somehow loosen the shackles. I had resided war-wearily at Bishopsthorpe for one year, and with this accommodation-related background safe and secure, it begged the question why was I revolving my life simply around lunchfulls of liver, egg and bacon, chips and peas, when I could be actively scheduling my time around proper restructuring. I could still guarantee that David would pop his head round my hotel door and proposition whether I would like my steak well done or medium rare, so it was a no loss risk

Fortunately there was a weather-beaten last outpost of Mental Health care, swaying gently on the breeze, no distance from Kirk's camera shop on Cobb's Corner. Through Dr Sess I was put on the register, and signed up for specialist mental health intervention and education to limit the regularity of hospital admissions, if that was possible. After two years I had been shown side entry into a proper mental health system. The Kirkdale Resource Centre issued all the hallmarks of a late Victorian institution, towering above the four stories of Bishopsthorpe, leaning forward on a gradient, like it was about to be swept out by the tide. Outwardly, it was well restored and had a mown front garden dissected by a wizard's pathway, arrowing up the incline to the intercom on the front door. Tentatively I rode up unchaperoned, leaving the mustang tied to the gatepost. It felt sad to be Hopalong Cassidy and not Billy the Kid anymore, but it was not humiliating to be officially seen by society as a mad client who goes to that weird place up the road that nobody talks about. What other necessary risks were on offer, apart from supposedly driving around in Sunshine Buses and being coaxed across a busy one-way street? If I found it unproductive I could always double back.

The paneled doors seemed to open automatically onto a dingy, derelict building full of past screams and bad omens.

There was no formal welcome, just a logbook to scribble my name in just to prove my existence. An unhelpful stairway ignored the newcomer as it wound straight up to all the therapeutic units, such as the cold and empty kitchen and a cozy meetings studio at the summit. I could hear the opening chorus to 'The Final Countdown' by Europe twisting its knuckles into the staff office to my immediate left, and a pretty blonde spluttered some protocol at me. I must sign the book in the lobby, and take an oath of anti-sexist and anti-racist behaviour, before breathing. Subdued by this insult to my intelligence, I was shown with pleasantries into the engine room of the asylum where smokers were sparsely puffing. The stale smoke bounced off the tangerine walls like rock pyrotechnics. It was unhealthy to be in this zoo, but I got on with it, to remove my winter coat, and stuff it jadedly on to the floor next to a cheap, flowery settee, where I parked. I didn't feel comfortable butting in to the general conversations of clients who ignored me. It wasn't that they were rude; it was just like making your presence felt at a party full of strangers.

The radio was punching out a dance track on Kiss FM, which stood head and shoulders below the black music of the seventies, and I noticed that it was so streamlined to the high ledge above that it was actually nailed on to it to prevent theft! Was this distrust warranted just because the crewmembers had a tendency to be ill? It certainly didn't follow David and Colin's controversial methods of yielding responsibility to people. At the heel of the sitting room was a tall, rectangular window that backed out on to a shabby garden that rose to the St Bartholomew's Church graveyard, which Pissarro thought picturesque enough to paint in the nineteenth century. It was likely that the sturdy green oaks and tuneful birds would have inspired him then, like they do today. After supplicating four mugs of tea which had joined the assemblage of empties on the low, square coffee table, I poached a copy of 'The Voice' newspaper which enlightened me about the racist mental health system. One or two of their journalists must have gone to UEA.

After thirty minutes of atrophy, I began to reminisce about the free-thinking and arbitration of the hostel, where it was time for the daily exchanges of Fifteen-to-One. I didn't go back to the Centre for another, painful year. Stable accommodation was not the only option for me to beat the tide, but still the best weapon to kick mental health problems. Bishopsthorpe cannot be underestimated in its solid basis for recovery, while vulnerable bedsitters at Kirkdale's Welfare Centre beat the smoke out of their chests. One rule and one rule only sufficed at the hostel where you were not privileged to put poor Dave through WWF wrestling on the telly. The clients were free to practice self-help in a way the Trust was keen to forbid. Colin even helped Donny install a photographic darkroom in his quarters, while Sahara practised her singing and the washing up very loudly in the kitchen. I almost could sense Liz's spirit gliding around in Dave's Renault, blasting out East 17 down a sleepy Kentish lane. It was Utopian - even without Summerslam.

By the fault of medication my wit was backfiring like a VW engine, and my sense of humour weakened. The old shrapnel wound of knowing my communicative qualities were unproven, slapped my face every time I spoke a corrupt and impaired language. I tried in vain to steady the sinking ship with blasts of forced humour and overt intellectual effort, that failed with every word I overdid. I was as unsubtle as an expletive in a Shakespearian sonnet, curdling the milk of human kindness within me. It hurt, pounding my broken heart with the precious articulation I could no longer fathom. The parts of my intellectual rebelliousness were oiled by wit and repartee, which translated to the page. Contrived ordinariness cannot be rebellion, and therefore wasn't me. I produced all the just conclusions of Salieri, as a Mozart who definitely had the talent which I alone could conceptualise. However instead of confounding the world I couldn't even confound our friends at Kirkdale. My legacy was the revolving door hospital statistic who needed constant supervision in the community. I had nothing to back up my certainty that I was something. I only mattered in the revitalising pastures of Bishopsthorpe, where the law of choice freed me from failure. Colin and Dave could not be blamed for watching Sheila 'Gobblecock' present the Norwegian weather forecast, deducing that finger pointing would only see anxiety cascade and self-esteem founder on the rocks.

13

Music was the only constant passion in my life, albeit dampened by the heavy drizzle of mental illness. My records were second-hand, which gave me quantity rather than quality. Terraplane mania had metamorphosed years previously into the standard rock formula known as 'Thunder', who had sold several million singles to me which had hauled them through the backdoor of the charts. Their global success richly merited their artistic credibility, but their conformity to a more regular and clichéd rock sound, sacrificed the spontaneity and spark of Terraplane. Remuneration had to come from somewhere, without which there would have been no future. Dutifully I bought all their records, but had I not been involved with the colour of Terraplane, the melancholia of Thunder I may have occasionally found dull. Their rebellious conservatism was simply Conservatism to which I could not comply and the relationship split like a divorce with the couple remaining good friends for the sake of the children. Thunder couldn't hold a stick of rock to the stick of dynamite that Terraplane once had been, and I became apathetic towards a stage show that creaked like Danny's old left knee. Had my illness of indifference migrated or were we all simply getting too old for rock 'n roll?

The massive gaping hole left behind by my love of this band, had to be filled by a thousand other stars collectively. In the sorry and lonely evenings and without June's soliciting, I consoled myself with T'Pau again to light the intellectual wasteland, and Ben Elton for a quick comic fix. Both were absolutely vital and medicinal to a suicidal state of mind. One night through my fog of gloom, Carol Decker's pure and beautiful voice seemed like the only light in a cold, dark and wintery world. It existed in the moment. As described, in recent times I have collected a decent selection of celebrity memorabilia whose photographs scale the back wall of this room and hang proudly from my kitchen shelves at the cost of much labour and love. One year I sent Carol a letter, who wrote back as enigmatically as an X-Files script. A month ago when I drew her attention to the reply at a the stage door of her West End play, she hustled passed me, oblivious to my little story. However I will never forget her glimmer of light in my total darkness.

Against all expectations, a solo artist was refilling the blind spot vacated by Terraplane. The Amadeus film was opening my ears to classical music, softly and subtlely. It may have not happened without Peter Shaffer's inspirational depiction of Mozart's music in words, but the soundtrack of the film crept up on me like the beginning of Mozart's Serenade for Thirteen Winds (3rd Movement). For both I and Salieri, the music started out "like a rusty old squeezebox", before culminating as "the very voice of God". Eventually, Shaffer's script didn't need to emphasize the music's meaning and Mozart just took me over, as if in total agreement with my mediocre counterpart, that "this was a music I had never heard before." Had I committed suicide during the earlier famine of my mental illness, I would have gone to heaven only to spin Terraplane records. This made staying alive a little more worthwhile and now I can dream that when I'm gone I might even play Piano Concerto Number 20, or Clarinet Concerto in A like Wolfgang Amadeus Mozart. When I consider the gentle spirit of his music to uplift all depressive moods, I may be able to accept that this demonstration of fate was perhaps more by design than chance.

All I knew was that in these dirty times that I had to prepare myself for hard labour to improve and never to give up. Rejection from June was never going to result in the ultimate showdown any more, but its complex clogged my arteries and its finality bruised my sore veins. Each day as I looked into my heart to see what I had done, a little more hope was gone. My faith was broken after all the determination to survive and stay in there for her, was rewarded by God with a slap in the face. There was no answer to the sorry shambles June had left behind, but to stay reclusively in Bishopsthorpe was not the answer for a winner to take all. Something had to be done to fight the lethargy and missing personality the drugs had criminally produced. It was thus decided by a Kirkdale Resource Centre majority that I should undergo some employment training which loosened my regular bowels to the extent that it warranted potty training. Working was simply not on the menu. I felt like I was being experimented on again to improve the Trust's image, who assumed that the greatest encounter I had in the world was against social prejudice. This attitude was no less prejudiced than the unlimited power they endowed a mad psychiatrist with to experiment with people's brains in the 'ECT Suite'. Their policies bypassed treatment en masse, for spineless, statistical selling points for which the government awarded gold stars. Everyone was happy except the patients.

I expected to come down on the Vocational Training and Assessment team, before they allayed my fears with quite reasonable expectations with no recourse to work forcibly. They had at once read between the Trust's demarcation lines between supposed success and failure, probably because if they hadn't they would have received no students. This enabled the course to be constructive without increasing tension about imminent work pressures looming on the near horizon. The 15-week course provided basic computer literacy, confidence building, assertiveness training and simple job interview techniques, as well as a discussion group on the pros and cons of the Mental Health Care system as facilitated by a user of the service. There were three project managers who couldn't have tried to sell the system any less, but maybe they were aware that they would have had a job convincing a schizophrenic that reality was no more than unreality! I respected their utter dedication and devotion to client welfare, and was surprised that I often exceeded the limits of my expectations without being knocked into shape, schoolmaster fashion. Unlike the statistically challenged rock face of political intrigue at the Trust, VTA dared to ask me with common sense about what I wanted and I began to get reacquainted with myself, which was an obvious goal of any therapeutic plan. I fought punctuality as a Clopixol cropper and survived, which unveiled the invaluable lesson of routine, all of which I achieved without going to work and getting ill. The VTA grounded some more fanciful ambitions temporarily, before reinstating a grain of enlightenment, and this hope did me proud.

At VTA there was nobody more informed about the services than the tutor who had incurred his own mental health difficulties. Gord' Carlile championed the rights of 'service users' of all backgrounds, doctrines and class without causing riots, and was a practical symbol for all those who regarded our social position as institutionalized. He was born in the wilderness as a spastic, who the doctors rigidly deemed would always be immobilized, and then he had led hundreds of young people out of the wilderness thereof, on foot, only pausing for medication at the halfway drinking hole. In divulging openly his personal diary of childhood abuse, foster care, care abuse, and family bereavement, I made him ten feet tall, despite his crablike but fully portable posture. I was impressed with the grace in which he shared his time with a world that he owed no favours to, and could justly have turned his back from. When I asked him for help it was forthcoming. There was no meanness in the expectation levels he tendered towards potential. By simple faith and hope in the student's realistic ambitions, he became proficient at saving many would-be victims, and this is what Gord' saw as his job. I clicked with Gord' intellectually after he had introduced me to the liquid form of his medication, and we were able to keep our objectivities from crossing the line of pessimism, for he taught me that "all people are dependant on each other." Without being stirred up in university dogma, I was guided liberally by his experience as a mental health lecturer by day, and as a worshipper of Phil Collins' 'Another Day In Paradise' on pub juke-boxes, by night.

He trained many care workers in his daily schedules, and innocently inquired one morning if I would like to assist him in an afternoon lecture in the Bexley Infirmary. When he saw me freeze with the anxiety of exposure, he dryly remarked that he only wanted somebody to turn over his flipchart, during the meeting. I reluctantly consented to the arrangement, rising somewhat unmagnificently to the occasion, but conforming to David's high-risk strategy.

It was my first visit to the hospital grounds in Bexley, which had a wholly unjustified reputation for brutality and high security. David used to escape to this archaic lieutenant of architecture for peace of mind, but only to visit a former resident of Bishopsthorpe who was too ill to live in the community, or as he sensitively put it "there for the rest of his natural." However, any jail looks rosier from the car-park. I actually went inside a small hut to assist with the lecture, which resembled an officer's mess. I didn't feel intimidated by an uneasy atmosphere, but by an expectant circle of vacant chairs, and a crowd of tea-drinking debaters, most of them female, looking butch enough to shred Gordon's male ego in about ten minutes. Gord' presently asked the predators to begin the group, and I calmly took over my post at the flip board. As he got the show on the road by introducing everybody to each other, including me, I recalled my university note making skills, which were soon adequately drafting down key words and relevant points in the discussion. It was as easy as selling pies in a mud factory, but my lack of exposure was perhaps being seized upon as a sign of inadequacy. As I lit a cigarette, lazily training my glance around the hospital grounds outside the window, Gordon lit the fuse to the spotlight on the world. His exact and deliberate words were: "And now over to Rob, who is going to give you his life-story." He smiled and then whispered like a true mate: "Just five minutes will do, Rob." A shadow was cast and my first utterance nearly blinked, "What, me?" With jaw below sea-level, akin to the scary television lights of Fifteen-to-One, which I came a creditable sixth in two years ago, I made a non confrontational speech which I doubt is still cherished in the minds of my audience. With sweaty hands and heart palpitations I ended my first and only public speaking engagement before Gordon rescued me by saying, "Thank you very much, Rob". After underscoring Gord's welcome return to the podium for a further twenty minutes, we took the money and ran, although I've lost his phone number. It's not in my jacket.. However, in the lobby afterwards, over tea and biscuits, I felt I had been listened to and treated as an equal of all the business-looking types, now making sense of my modest account of myself. However, after a celebratory Stella with Gordon in a non ring fenced establishment, the daylight dawned on me that the game of Happy Families was just a sham, for it was more like a rifle range and we weren't the ones holding the blindfolds. They still saw themselves as the professionals. Well I did.

1995 was the year of my fulfillment, when all the loose ends to my life knitted together into a ball of string. The punishment of medication was unrelenting, as was the pain and dismal content of my psyche. The golden path that trickled like a camel nursing itself through the eye of a needle, was littered with tripwire. However, the size of each tiny step forward didn't matter alongside the adherence to direction. Those that signposted the farewell from danger were a various chocolate assortment of good and semi-good, but profoundly involved in my person. I was dying inside from the tip of my mute tongue to the nerve endings on my swollen feet. I had already failed in the counseling arena after the six short weeks it took to galvanize volcanic matter However, I told Dr Sess that I would like one further chance, while his gaggle of young female nurses drooled over his imperious decision. I clarified that I wanted to talk through the eight years of hell with a woman counselor if I could get the NHS out of bed. Sess surprised me by not circumnavigating me around to Hecate's office, and awarding an instant and reasonable judgment in my favour. He commented that he could fix me up with a newly promoted female psychologist who had uprooted from Farnborough Hospital, near Bromley, to a new post in the Lewisham and Guy's Mental Health Trust. This meant fortunately that she could be teamed with the Kirkdale Resource Centre. This coincidence was fortunate enough to please me, and I left him to continue his wenching.

I took up the slack in a small matter of two weeks, which defied the dense gravitational pull of red tape in the Mental Health system, remarkably. I was tossed through the Kirkdale Resource Centre shop window once more, signed the book, avoided the plumes of smoke, and trod the staircase for the very first time, past a perennially devoid kitchen, to a tinderbox counseling room the size of a lift. There were two easy red chairs in this room whose window looked down exhaustively at the rain-washed streets I had eluded. On the left was a cheap, wooden bookcase with a lone book about art therapy lying in state at half-mast, which seemed to swamp any spare space, and to the right, was a crusty old radiator pumping out heat.

I was wheezing from the climb, but began to breathe more regularly when she greeted me with a lopsided smile and a quietly confident air of knowing. I had not dressed for the occasion very well, but she was gowned immaculately and not ostentatiously, like she was conference bound. Sitting about four feet away, she introduced herself as one, Bessie Harris. I had to divert my attention away momentarily to her slender ring finger, and yes she was. Her misty blue eyes did not flinch away from me, and were already tuned in to her waiting-game style, emphasizing the dual responsibilities of counseling. She would interject soundly, but it was clear from the tilt of her wispy head that her ears were pinned on what I wanted to say. Rather than drop-dead gorgeous she was unconventionally pretty. Her voice was silky, and soothingly pitched, but her unassuming gait never rose imperialistically. I was interested by this Mini being pushed by a Ferrari engine. My only reservations on first impression, was that she might be nosy or gossipy, but I assume that a counsellor should be to get to the truth through the blind alley of conversation. She struck me like Agatha Christie's old spinster sleuth, Jane Marple. Both possessed an instinct for human nature, and were not as frail and innocent as their modesty suggested.

In our first session, she spoke approximately twice in one hour, but her attention to my guilty outpouring were intense. It felt good to be talking about the clinical dismissal Junie had broken me with, and how my secret writing talent had not impressed, beyond the onset of my illness on that fateful night, many years ago. Underneath I was asking her to heal my pain, and if she couldn't undo that, then patience would suffice. One session per week was planned and open to me for as long as I needed her help, or until the Trust relocated her to the Kremlin. I feared justifiably that speed was of the essence in this treatment, despite her sincere promises that Hecate could never set her hypodermics on my manhood again. After week one, the world had not shifted and if it had I wouldn't be the water-fetcher or soil-tiller. However, as I descended the staircase and exited to the camera shop some hundred yards away, I became aware of a sudden burst of spiritual healing running down my soul path, predicting or prophesying no detailed promises or bargains to be had, but allowing for a sense of calm, to signify a better road.

The plot had moved forward from my three pivotal and successful years in the Bishopsthorpe establishment. I had no pressing need to play scrabble every night while David would devilishly fumble around in the bag for blank tiles. The token Slimfast diets with Dave were not working, particularly after the evening steak and chips cooked to any specifications of rare, medium or well done. I was also still craving for the silliness of the WWF. Something had to give like independent accommodation, which I would never dare to organize without David and Colin's permission, or their company's care in the community networks. I knew that part of the deal at the hostel was to prepare a sound platform for take-off into independent-living if it was felt necessary by a client wishing to climb his ladder of responsibilities. The other option was to stay put in a comfortable, clean and safe environment with no duress to move on, which was a challenge I had comprehensively exhausted. It was another risk. Junie was still playing tragically on my mind, and I was still playing head games, half expecting her to change her mind and reveal herself. I am ashamed to announce that my overriding reason for change was to impress her with the luxury of a self-made flat. Despite David's cognitive thinking and virtual capacity to be a mind-reader, nobody touted these real but ridiculous thought-patterns, although sound and whispered objections were relayed. I had to show them that my commitment was serious so I made contact with a social worker in the Forest Hill social services department, glancing over my shoulder at the impressions this action left on the two hostel proprietors. I never intended to forge ahead without them, but I had to convince them that I was serious of burning my boats if necessary to dwell under a banner of social welfare. After all the dedication, fraternization, tears and laughter, this would not be an appropriate conclusion for either party, and it did the trick. Being entrepreneurial anyway, David and Colin were not thick enough to pass up the opportunity of making a few quid. It was a question however, of whose reservations was more guaranteed; theirs or the bank manager.

New faces came to captain the Bishopsthorpe ship to enable Colin and Dave some recreation and to spare us the thrice weekly yawns of Eastenders and The Bill. Considering the monotonous patterns of daily schedules and the tight fit of familiar household veterans, their willpower, even to sleep on the two main sofas night after night, needed extending. I could switch off from displeasing antics in the joy of my own space, but David and Colin were pretty much confined to one room, together, for three wearying years.

Most of the pubs in Sydenham were naff which settled well with Colin's pessimism. He was a pleasant man who sank pretty rapidly every time he took up the easel. His intentions pointed to the soon to be improved attic, where he could cook up an Old Master, before cutting off his left ear. The only problem was that by tea-time, he had only enough faith left to cook up a vegetable curry, which he stirred like the incessant doubt going round and round in his head. However, his unheralded stroke of genius was to challenge Amber and Ilona to friendly games of pool in the Golden Lion.

Their names conjured images of the two West Indian night-nurses who had cruelly and blatantly poked scorn at their broken, pathetic and out of reach patient at 5am in Great Yarmouth's infirmary. Instead, when pressed, Colin divulged forlornly and hopelessly "they were more like models." The wiping of his steamed up glasses once more, yielded an impressive truth. I learnt that they had both been invited for weekend shifts on the premise that for the first time, they had not deemed a Colin a cowboy when he had revealed what he did for a living at an unregulated hostel. Unbelievably they were studying psychiatry at university, and it also helped that they could scoop extra proceeds from Colin's lamentable wages over the green baize. Drinking like fish was simply the cherry on the cake.

Weekday work was also delegated conditionally to Jo, a Northamptonshire traffic warden with a nutty sense of humour, which made her a unique but prize acquisition. If the two psychiatric students should be addressed as models then it would be appropriate to describe Jo as a role model, perfectly attired, punctual and without fault. As soon as she was interviewed the list of other candidates was shredded. I liked what I saw immediately, and when consulted about her appointment, I backed Dave and Colin one hundred percent. The other significant inclusion in the team was a caring mother of three teenage daughters, who had infinitely more experience in employment than the cleaning and cooking tasks she was given. Carol unexpectedly made light work of her duties and brought a sensitive presence to the hostel, which perhaps the others did not inspire. She was capable of working her back off for those she cared for either at home or in homes, and was thus a brilliant candidate to be a mental health worker and let David and Colin have a little more time off.

However, excitement was at fever pitch, with the two young girls ready to figure. Wanting and needing a girlfriend, made every potential chance into a beauty. It was possible that my vulnerability to a sweet natured woman like Bessie had built her up too far in my estimation, for example, although she had enough magnetism for an admirer to build up an electric field of intensity. However when I clocked the first of the lovelies nervously leaning forward over the edge of the sofa one Saturday morning, it was like Marc Anthony meeting Cleopatra. She was lean, with symmetrically cupped cheekbones and her lips were an achingly sweet, bright red that pouted into a completely unpretentious smile that loved the universe. Her face and solid stream of auburn hair could have scuppered the Armada. However, I challenge anybody who encounters Ilona to not be stunned by her compassionate eyes, which seem to silence the panic of the world with an extraordinary beauty. What else could a thirsty man want, when she had a stretch of long legs, and a fit, feminine frame, as well? Even a gentle spirit seemed to clothe her skin, like a satin bridal gown. There was no more inwardly beautiful soul to ever have graced our hostel and that was just for starters. By one o'clock she even worked out the temperamental deep fat fryer, to serve up a pretty mean omelette and chips for our lunch.

That Saturday the sun must have shone on my rehabilitation like never before. Ilona was a class act, but I still couldn't believe Colin's dismal recommendations twice in a row. After a two hour night's kip, the doorway woke me on the stroke of ten, and I eagerly slipped on a dirty pair of Bermuda shorts to assess our newest recruit. I was groomed in modesty, with bags under my sleep-filled eyes, and twenty-something whiskers falling from my runny nose. I fixed a morning coffee, and still squinting from the Sunday daylight, I stumbled heavily into a half-built conservatory that Colin had single-handedly constructed all Summer long, to assuage the heartache of another more difficult kind of canvass. He politely introduced me to his friend with a predictable smirk as my tongue unrolled itself to the deck for the seven hundred and sixty eighth time in twenty-four hours. This was Amber and it took her twenty four seconds to assert that I should change out of my dirty trousers, like she was dressing a salad. I had been dismissed with keen and reproachful eyes like cannon fodder. I took no offence spun round on the back foot, and coughed out a tense giggle. By lunchtime, I had even been fined one roast potato from an exquisite Sunday dinner, for needlessly trying to banter with her, but all was in good humour. While most men would have lowered their jackets into a puddle for her to walk upon, I somehow became involved in losing duels with Amber that were stimulating for me, and full of sentiment. Colin could not have described his heroine any more clearly. She was an inch or two shorter than Ilona, with a physique like a piece of string and the envy of most cat walkers. Her abundant golden hair was unbleached and her face absolutely radiant. She was hot property, and she had a personality to match. I hastily adjudicated that most of her men would be official candidates for a sleeper hold perfected by some of the WWF wrestlers I was not allowed to watch any more. Amber had all the rapid fire of Rowdy Roddy Piper, when she wasn't the delicate femininity of his manager, Miss Elizabeth.

I couldn't have prayed for two nicer or more dedicated people to watch out for me than these two kids and they grasped the principles and demands of mental health care as surely as anybody still training ever could. They were so miraculous that I concluded that they were angels sent from above, whose purpose on the Earth was to feed and clothe the sick and hungry. However, for these early weekends in their career it became apparent that they were exclusively working for me. They were that special that even I reevaluated my stance on God.

The key to that lock was turned by the next new client, who had been kicked out of the Salvation Army for alcohol abuse. Their loss was my gain however, when he unrolled his gift for Knowledge, which could not be found in any scripture or religious formality. Rod Deaver was a stern looking forty seven year old, with the disposition of a pre war Hollywood cad. He even had the Errol Flynn moustache, and wore gun slinging two piece suits, bought laudably, round the corner from the Oxfam shop I ended up working in. He always tended to be serious, but never intellectually overbearing, but whenever he spoke from his mind, the world listened intently.

God still frightened me intensely, but His instrument was not intimidating in the least. Rod moved into one of the first floor rooms and he impressed me by the lack of mess that featured so prominently in all the other clients' dens. While I was still burdened with unanswered and just questions, his only peace of mind permutated in his religion. Therefore he became a spiritual teacher and guide, and the anchor weight between God and the bottom of the deep blue sea. The only paradox that could undo my scriptural indoctrination at university, was from sound non-Biblical spirituality, and Rod had the very validity because he had never learnt to read or write. It was the most adequate solution to a life of dangerous and non-scientific evaluations of God. Roddy could explain in layman's terms the right prescription for a schizophrenic distortion of Biblical fantasies, by calling upon his reliable Knowledge to whitewash the dirt sprayed in my face by ecclesiastics. His meritorious observations pulled my face out of the Good Book as he fed me common sense, that religious passages had made me doubt. If only God were like this.

The exodus from the Bishopsthorpe hostel to new premises at the end of the street was not stressful, because Dave and Colin were there to smoothly assist. I reveled in my wonderful achievement, and for the first two days of occupation, I polished meticulously the grotesque wooden furniture Dave had pulled out of his secret lock-up, once used by the makers of Steptoe and Son. It was a spacious one bedroom flat, with more potential in the sunlit sleeping quarters, than in the murkier pond of the sitting room to be fair, but just to be here was more than enough, for a man biting his hundred and seventeenth cherry. I could say I did it for Junie's love and that she could at last respect her fallen hero, but it also proved that at twenty-seven years of age, and nine years of schizophrenia, I had become somebody. I could search with Bessie's expertise for the dead soul of that man, and maybe wake up one day, happy to be alive in his hands. Bess and I were optimistic about what we were working for.

After a few discussions, Carol was appointed to oversee the new accommodation-related mess and to lift the lingering smog of 'soiled clothes' that littered all four floors. After the first grandiose days of contented honeymoon, the 'rotation' of clothes had lost its verve. She popped along to the flat every Wednesday for an hour, to save my life fleetingly from the piles of dishes and the empty pizza boxes and beer bottles that rose to the ceiling like the ensuing cash-flow crisis to pay for them. I had not mastered the routine of supermarket shopping, and paying bills on time, and I felt the pinch of self-determination. Rod had hinted that life was "not a game."

14

Nobody becomes a hero without endeavour or by struggling to overcome the mistakes of one's ignorance. One distant day, the leaning on support workers would eventually end, like being set adrift on a raft at sea, with only my hands to wrestle high winds and repairs. I have seen very little of David and Colin and 'the family' since such contingencies beckoned wildly about two years ago, but now these achievements and labours are rich enough for all to see in my home, from which I have constructed a palace. When I invite guests into my flat I am sharing my inner pride at overcoming the odds of survival all starting from the wickedness of UEA. The sprawl of gadgets and toys simply manifests as the outpouring of care I have shown myself. If David and Colin entered, I would want them to be proud about what their flat says about them, and how I regard myself, not simply that it is overflowing with extraordinary eccentricity.

Rod always exposed the light on Biblical shortcomings. He believed in prayer but refreshingly, told me not to have too much faith. "Too much faith is no good", confounded much established gospel rhetoric, which encourages too much faith. I had abandoned prayer when Paul had been killed in the road accident in 1978, the scarring of which, according to Bess was "permanent". After my prayers for his life had been tossed aside, I refused any more chances for God to rub my nose in it. Roddy taught me however, that "you've got to know how to pray", and sometimes you just do. It simply comes down to whether you can put together the right words and phrases into the correct order, or you can't. It doesn't mean God will listen, but it doesn't really matter, so long as the articulation tallies. Not trusting the counselor helped, because in picking careful and proper sentence structures to evade the truth, I reckoned she would have to second guess all the time whether I needed further Depixol. Consequently I became an able communicator for a while, and with my Nemesis.

Soon without warning (or asking) I received a Gift of my own. A white, spiritual mist seemed to purvey beneath my arms and legs, and along my torso, enabling even more insight into the world besides prayer. Roddie instinctively adjudged that I had "so much fickin' knowledge now", just so I understood that this wasn't a ridiculous flare-up of schizophrenia again. To underline this newfound headway, Bessie rang David quite against the grain of her aloof principles, to confirm how pleased she was with my abundant insight. I believe that Rod's gift had filled a gap in my spirituality and been passed on, and for many months he and I, communicated on a similar frequency and higher plane.

Shortly other spiritual gifts developed out of my template of Knowledge. I became able to see into a world of Philosophy, Psychology and Wisdom as each formidable talent landed like a spotlight on my head chakra from above. The gap between Bessie's unblocked, reasoning powers and my fuzzy, medication-rabbled catatonic prison must have narrowed, because I could only candidly and cheekily point out to her one day, that "it feels like I'm counseling you!"

She never engaged in the complexities of war very enthusiastically, although she was never a pushover. With pencil in hand, and in lethal concentration, she would throw another baffling question at me and bring me back into line. Her calculating eyes alone could pierce the shenanigans of any miscreant as quickly as the bawling and screaming of a sergeant-major. The more she puzzled me, the deeper my affection for her, which caused several, inevitable hiccups. Her dirty body was positively corrupting, and there it reclined just feet away from its predator once a week for three slobbering years. Fortunately her compelling mind hid her true personality, emotional discharge, and personal life from my active prurience, to keep the sessions, sweet and clean, and sensationally productive for my balance of ill-health.

The new duty psychiatrist, Dr Johnny Coogan, pulled no punches in describing her as "fantastic" and Rod spotted that I needed to have "faith and confidence" in someone, and not necessarily a God which was cheering. Paradoxically, the less Bessie spoke the less I feared her and trusted she didn't actively enjoy expelling patients to Hither Green like a whole host of Hatecrimes would have been inclined to do. She became confidant to my growing confidence in bridging the gap between the system over there and the patient under here. There was absolutely no punishment in honestly describing the misery I felt.

For more sessions than I can remember, I simply blurted out the unrequited trauma regarding Junie. Bess patiently never rammed any opinion down my throat, until one day she could have knocked me down with a feather, when she leant forward in her chair, conferring compassionately that "I don't see her hurting." In silence I grappled with the gravity of this unstoppable argument. The truth was brought home. Unlike my ex-sweetheart, Bessie fearlessly wanted to hear the details of my gruesome story between the university years. I dropped the hampered hamminess, and concentrated on restoring my resources, being ever strengthened by a wave of straight-laced candour. The biggest test came when I thought that TV stars might be relaying coded messages and instructions for me to act on. Although I was fully cognizant this time of the unwelcome intrusion of my schizophrenia, I had to tell somebody pretty quickly. Bess stood back and rearranged the downward spiral of a distorted psyche instantly. Her invaluable training softened the blow to be "ideas of reference" a term applied to a variable of schizophrenia. There was no impetus to obey these implications, just to ride with the understanding that they couldn't harm me. I ended the session by cautiously throwing in the kitchen sink and it swam. I informed Bessie that I thought it was Julia Roberts who was offering the most glaringly obvious advice, and what should I do? Unstirred and unemotional to the content, Bess passed a baffling conjuring trick, that totally made up for the lost time imposed by initial distrust. She said: "That must be very comforting". After the delay of sparring, our counseling relationship lanced all aspects of my depression without realizing quite how it had been done. Coogan was right. I knew in my head beyond all doubt that she was the best thing that ever happened to me, but perhaps more significantly, I knew inside that she was the only person who had ever loved me, and the only person I had ever loved.

Any psychologist will determine that love comes in many forms and shapes. I felt no love for Bess and yet I knew I loved her. Was this type of love so different and alluring that it neutralized the raging passion for June, as inconsequential? Why could this weird lady who had unloaded zero emotional feedback while often looking at my feet or out of the window to assess me, possess more meaning to her love, than even my parents? There was also a tangible and real, one-way love swimming inside me over Amber. Was that not what I had been needing?

She was my only link to actual emotion, probably because her natural love, compelled mine to break out from my darkened and derelict tomb. If I dared to be honest, I loved her forever, and it validated my good person with a feeling to give.

It was strangely true that I was in the somewhat unenviable position (some would say enviable) of being totally besotted and rocked to my foundations by three separate women, in the same moment. It was exhausting just to rotate Amber, Ilona and Bess's naked fantasies through my excited lust, but it was equally frustrating that they had no romantic sympathies towards me. Bessie was decent enough to "really respect the polite way" I brought my sensualities to her attention, and she was kind enough to add that she was "not without feelings for you either", before jamming the slightly ajar door with my case notes.

I wanted one more try to feel and perform sexually by finally dropping medication. In the past, even in respect to the crises, the normal sexual animal had always been restored after a minimum of five missed doses. This allowed my natural confidence with women to spiral, albeit at the short-term expense of lucidity. Although I respected Bess's boundaries, I couldn't let any hope of attracting either of the two girls pass me by. Without close contact or human touch for most of my adult life, I was irretrievably lonely if just for a caressing female hand.

Dr Coogan was probably the only decent consultant psychiatrist to ever work in the London Borough of Lewisham, and in true impish style he had resigned a healthy stipend in the military to work, more with court cases than court martials. After repeated experimentation by deafened psychiatrists on my organs and bowels, I trusted him initially less than a Jew trusts a Palestinian sex-case. It was his call to undo prejudicial wrongs and work in progress previously inflicted on me by his profession, and he shouldered his steepling burden with dignified commitment. His gradual reversal of the traditional tide of suspicion that accompanies a new appointment was so major that it was unheard of. I reversed his name fondly to Major John. He was a straight man without the gusto of military discipline, and he could relay a sense of humour through dark, twinkling eyes, more like an effigy of Sergeant Bilko, than a schizophrenic analyst. I heard he was a devout Roman Catholic which surprised me, because I could read his blessed judgments beautifully. Like Bess, he was nobody's fool and a military hard nut.

To barter at his level one had to be right on one's guard, and with my abundance of spirituality I elucidated reasonably, that I wanted to forfeit my medication to empower the obedience of my body again. Coogan's sugary response was thought provoking to put it mildly: "Is that wise?" I didn't really know if it was wise, and only considered the numerous outcomes. How did I really know what could result from this dramatic change of direction? My determined decision however, would not be reversed at this late hour for any sound conjecture, and he gave in, gesticulating, "Alright Robert, you win!"

If I could detox from the deadly daily drug like never before, I could still be the eighteen year old beauty even 'he' had long ceased to be. Without medication blocking my resources, I could fulfill my vast earning potential and still be in the limelight as a writer of comedies or plays for either stage or screen. I wanted to prove to those like Ilona who had faithfully insisted that all my talent was still animate, that I was the genuine article and not boasting from my posterior. My wit and sense of humour would no longer be agonizingly corroded from the energy sources in my solar plexus and feet that sheltered the entire central nervous system. Perhaps the girls might notice me eating an ice-cream in the park, and not disdainfully accelerate past my medication-buffeted body. I had nothing but everything to lose. Was it one risk too far? The deal was clinched however, when Amber rounded angrily on me to ask if I preferred visual hallucinations to impotence. I had been impotent so long, that I didn't think she needed an acknowledgement.

Without warning almost one week later, I wrote my first poem. The gift spotlighted my head chakra from above like before. After ten pulsating years of mediocrity, I suddenly possessed a device that was entirely switched in its infinity. The day was too unexceptional to note down, but one day it might be recorded as my finest hour. The power to unburden all past agonizing riddles in a creative milieu, multiplied each sacred hour for Bessie and I to dwell upon. The gift expressed an inner content which had ridden all the blows of mental hell, and it was highly literate, with humour, surrealism, and rhythmic verse, that I confess, I was not responsible for alone. Artistic titles seemed to flash into my head, as a higher power held my hand dragging a pen across a blank page into beautiful wordplay. From flat to breathlessly recharged batteries, I concocted one poem per day, giving me complete, therapeutic fulfillment. Like Arthur I had seen my kingdom destroyed only to sink to my knees in thanksgiving, and drink from the Holy Grail again. The time had come. I wrote copiously about Bess and my brace of angels, who were kind enough to admire my sentiments about them, and they encouraged me to keep the cold tap running despite it encroaching a little into their professional washbasin. Poetry worked like a charm and gave me charm, and for the first moment since I had been slapped on necessary benefits, I felt my jaw move while I talked. I was a respectable commentator in a competitive, social workplace.

The final link to the chain was the shiny gemstone. Stuffed up my jumper was ten years of the most hideous suffering the world has ever seen, like it was a ten foot genie, caged in

Aladdin's lamp. I had tried to force this suicidal energy out on to the confessional altar, through wasted prayer and exhibitions of shame. None of it washed with an unchanging and miserly God. I was climbing the rock face inside the white-hot pits of Krakatoa. I had already chalked a lot of grief and unfounded guilt onto the blackboard slate, which Bessie had wiped clean for me. However, traces of chalk dust still clogged my airstream like a smoking casualty's lungs. I didn't own a CD player because of a strong affiliation to the vinyl years, but I was musically accessible enough to have songs and tunes whistling round my ears all day. That breakthrough day was no different when I spent my last pound on Phil Collins 'But Seriously' album, that contained Gord's favourite track 'Another Day In Paradise'. There was a middle ground that Bess and David had urged me to find, without ever conferring and I suppose with a love of rock and classical music, the brass explosion and lonesome heartbeats of Phil Collins filled the void aptly. While Thunder had cooled down, I had headhunted every worthy successor, but found no artist to shift my confirmed bias. Musically I was treading water, like the tiresome boy band phenomenon of the 1990s. I even investigated Roger Whittaker with just a subtle air of non-conformism, and quite rightly won the accolade for worst performer seen live, by Andy's work mates. It was the following morning that was meant to be exciting with a planned meeting with Bess. Today, had been the least dramatic day of my unexceptional life with an unadventurous early night planned, listening to music on an old, one pound cassette, and, me. That evening two minutes before the stroke of ten, as the tape reached the climax of side two, with my legs dangling over the two-seater sofa, and my eyes glazed with sleep, a miracle moved the world. An avalanche of Amazonian rain engulfed both Americas. I cried reservoirs with tears the size of bouncing bombs like I was swimming in my own busted dam. There was an indefinable holy trinity in my messy, and ragged living room, which was, myself, Bessie's spirit and what I can only deduce as the God I should have known. It was understandable that I hadn't really ascertained beneath the wailing commotion, that it was really the peace, serenity and sincerity of Phil Collins' music that had sensationally drawn a picture of a new dawn for me and reached inside to every level of my lifetime's journey through the cesspit of Hell. The record playing was 'Father to Son' and its beautiful simplicity seemed to stretch far beyond ordinary time and space. It had to, to reach me. After the shock had worn off, I played back the lyrics to the song in my mind, thus:

'Somewhere down the road, you're gonna find a place.

It seems so far but it never is.

And you won't need to stay, but you might lose your strength on the way.

Sometimes you may feel you're the only one

'Cos all the things you thought were safe, oh now they're gone.

But you won't be alone, 'cos I'll be here to carry you along

Watching you till all the work is done.

And when you find your heart, you'd better run with it,

'Cos when she comes along, she could be breaking it.

You know there's nothing wrong, you're learning to be strong, don't look back.

And she may soon be gone, so don't look back.

She's not the only one remember that.

If your heart is beating fast then you know she's right.

If you don't know what to say well that's alright.

If you don't know what to do

Remember she is just as scared as you.

Don't be shy even when it hurts to say,

Remember, you're gonna get hurt someday anyway.
Then you must lift your head and keep it there,
Remember what I said.
I'll always be with you don't forget.
Just look over your shoulder I'll be there,
Oh..
If you look behind you, I will be there.
If you look behind you, I will be there.

Was this a monumental idea of reference, with my schizophrenia wishing an idealized reality with its magic wand? Or was it the moment the chain was broken with the light of fortune finally eclipsing the massive black hole I had been staring into? Just whose voice had beckoned me on with such enchantment? Bess had always mused that I "didn't have to know why." but it was her love that seemed to have reached me. The counselor I so desired had strung all these magnificent sentences together for me from her heart. I know that my schizophrenia may be distorting the truth, but I am not exaggerating the personal interpretation that was stuck on to the facts in that one famous moment. There was no promise of jam tomorrow in the song just an innocent line that sang to me: "You're OK, you're alright, you made it."

I repeatedly rewound the tape all nightlong to be sure of my finding and each time I cried buckets until the well was dried by sleep. Typically in the morning, I theorized intellectually about what had happened but it offered me no new answers to my ancient questions. Why had this happened now and not at university where my imploded silence needed to speak through tears to the entire audience of undergraduates? Why had God made this suffering last forever, when He could have got me to listen to this cassette any time since 1989? And what was the point of all that fetching church music.

Once, someone somewhere had seized my inner spirit in one of our counseling sessions and spoke through me. I exasperated in a holy, holler, hotter than Bessie that "I wish you had been there" for my one-man holocaust at UEA. Maybe I couldn't redesign fate for myself then and had to wait until now for this tender teacher to grace me. When I had revived my weeping, rouged countenance I turned up for the truly fated counseling slot the next day a model of composure. The fits of tears was a passing matter of no consequence! However it was timely that I could discuss straightforwardly last night's dream with the governess of my heroic fortune. However as I sagged along past Kirk's Cameras, I was still at it, and ruing my permanently empty Kleenex box.

When I hit the Kirkdale Centre, Bessie promptly hustled me upstairs to our tiny box-room, before I had even the breath left to wolf-whistle at her wiggling behind. She might have already assessed me then as I held on up the steep hill, as being a little agitated or "tearful". We sat opposite each other ready to start and I just let her have it. My avalanche of last night's tears exploded again like the alien in John Hurt's tummy. There was not a chance in hell of reciprocating the steely aloofness that was assessing my desolate overflow. Both unmoved and relaxed without even a sip of cool water, she gently assented after I had finished blubbing for the time being that "You're feeling tearful"! It was so nice of her, that by then my eyes just accumulated more snow. Salieri had his fitting lacrymosa with just as many tears as he required, neither more nor less.

God was fated to have one last gasp attempt to drive me off the sane and rational road to recovery. I was living with my illness now, and was moderately accepting its debilitation. I agreed fully with Dave's supposition that the medication robbed the illness of taking over the personality and that it was my "responsibility" to keep them separate. If I couldn't trust

Dave by now, I could still trust his insight. However since I had discarded the Risperidone for the very last time, a hospital admission was farcically becoming touch and go. Everybody knew it, and I knew it, except I couldn't concede defeat to it. I began to incur short-term memory lapses, frighteningly forgetting where I had just been, and how I could reach desired destinations. My concentration also diminished. At the Kirkdale Centre's drop-in, which I now frequently attended, I was among the usual crew in the sitting room, when an uncontrollable urge came over me to stare into the eyes of Lady Diana, regaling in one of the left-wing newspapers on the coffee table. As I stared the face changed and became alive and started snarling at me. I was fully aware that I was hallucinating, but unwilling to sideline my hasty ambitions with the medication. I had put the whole support network on full alert, and next time it was Bess's turn to become a visual cropper. As we debated the recent recriminations in our next session I saw her head turn into an apple, which didn't seem to ruffle a single implacable hair. I thought immediately that my admission would scold my gentle neighbour, but not a bit of it; she had read my anxiety riposted vigorously that she, "was in no way feeling threatened." I always ensured I took my medication before meeting Bess because I respected her role as a mother of two as much as she was my judge and jury, and I didn't want ludicrous behaviour to topple that. On this occasion therefore, I coolly pulled out a tablet, and addressed my calm counselor that I was going to take it from its silver pouch and swallow it. Bess just nodded in a more enthusiastic fashion than I was used to, and serenely argued an emphatic "yes."

However, it had now became so bleak that I couldn't see even the most worryingly obvious warning signs. Later that same afternoon while I was deliberately diverting my gaze from Diana's photograph in the paper, Bess beckoned me over from the sitting room doorway. She declared that she had fixed me up to see Dr Coogan with the slim hope he might offer me some rope. I declined the offer playfully, and said: "I would like to see him, but first let's see him sweat." Then for the first day in living memory Bess just about lost her rag and snapped with the ferocity of a Verdi Requiem: "Look Rob, I'm so bloody scared you're going to end up in hospital." However, in the nicest eyes I shall ever visit was a look I know I'll never forget. It was alive with feeling and caring intensity. I knew beyond doubt that she was on my side above anybody, which unfortunately at this late stage of affairs did not include Dr Coogan. He could not stem the flow of hallucinations either and when he sat me down for a few rude truths I saw him mutate into Ronnie Barker. However, because he could see the futility of the situation before I did, he left me with one really useful clue for what I should be like, when I leave the next inevitable coma of hospital supervision. Instead of one of Dr Sess's low blows about the seriousness of my condition, Major Tom quipped nicely "You have two fabulous gifts of Empathy and Sensitivity." It was food for thought even then, because after all those years ago in the UEA coffee shop I had recently become aware that I did slant towards Encouragement, without ever really knowing it. This time I took on board what Coogan was saying before it took another ten years to verify another shrewd observation. I had been blind to the lesson that some people can read others better than they could read themselves. However, I was so far gone by now that I couldn't concentrate on my true friends' and carers' compassionate dictums before I forgot them.

15

David and Colin wanted me back in Hither Green, and every morning Colin had me on the phone to check I had made it safely through the night. Unfortunately I was now interpreting his goodwill as being pestered, and Rod inflamed the situation by jealously vilifying Colin for every tenth lager he popped. Briefly, it turned ugly against someone who had always gone out of his way to care for me. I listened to Rodney too eagerly, hanging on the edge of his gift for perfect truth. However in the cool light of day his resources only betrayed a personal axe to grind with the truth, not for it. I was almost picked up by the 202 bus on its way to Hither Green, when he decided that "Colin is going to ruin your life and put you in hospital." There was no way out of God's predestination, and I became utterly wild at the terror of more forced injections and even more suicidal impotence. David, on the other hand, was not moved to Rod's bitter barking, which he described as being "picked up over time from church meetings." He replaced Carol in her decontamination duties to oversee the imminent admission, and, because Rod described him as "the greatest man that ever lived, I raised no resistance. When he let himself in at a tacit hour to catch me unguarded, the "soiled clothes" spread-eagled from here to Elephant and Castle had run out of floor space. There was even a soggy pile stacked up to the ceiling that I had just dumped straight from the washing machine. We traded insults which was always fun, with typically neither one of us willing to back down. I ordered him to leave the flat I occupied on behalf of his money, with Dave continuing to lecture me. Finally after twenty minutes the storm blew itself out and in a spooky coincidence he looked at me with the exact same caring intensity that had registered in Bessie's eye just twenty-four hours ago. I know now that if this unforgettable warning sign should ever repeat then I will immediately take my tablets, even if it means handing the lash to Hecate.

In the end I admitted myself with inches to spare, recalling Dave's less hostile advice three years ago, to "take the pills, avoid a Section Three, and be out in a couple of days." My complete disintegration however had been a close call, and it took more than a weekend to recapture my strength and mental coherency. I arrived at the unsafe sentence that I was 'the beast' in the Book of Revelations, because I had dared to speak up to a priest about it, thereby incurring a junk load of God's Plagues and Curses. I was too scared to discredit His avenging wrath against me, and it felt necessary to protect the universe from the unhappy traitor I was, by killing myself. As I lay dormant and delusional in my asylum bed, I conceptualized the feeling that I was being flattened by all His earth and sky, and the extent of the whole ocean. God could rebuild a better world with the devil gone, so I made a puckish, but ultimately feckless suicide bid in the tin bath at the end of the corridor. As I lowered my head beneath the steaming waters of the half-empty bath, my ears heard the shouts of Hell's demons as they pulled me down to God's holy cavern for sinners and non-believers. The end was nigh. Fortunately there was an escape clause in my unsigned contract on stand-by. One of my favourite nurses put her head round the door more out of opportunism than voyeurism, and gently whisked me out by the scruff of my neck, and almost disbelievingly asked me what I had been doing.

To arrive on the scene of the crime corresponds to the notion that this just wasn't my time to die. Did this ironic twist of fate tally with the philosophy, that I was the bloke that God liked to crush like peppercorns? Maybe He had simply rescued me because I deserved a break, and some help for a change. Maybe it was because I was a "good person", according to Bess. And maybe it was because one of the alcoholic patients had excitedly decided I was Jesus and I had some Holy retribution to enact. All the usual Samaritans came by to the hospital to mend their friend, before being fit and well enough to leave.

However a mystery man enrolled in my associations, who came to offer sympathy to the patients from a meaningful light. He was a Muslim ecumenical, dressed like Bin Laden before he emigrated to Southern California to be a deckchair attendant. I had seen him on previous admissions literally holding the hand of the sick and taking their side like no doctor. He was always very friendly, and had a common man's twinkle in his eyes, as if he knew instinctively the solution that the patient beside him was searching for. One day near remission, we spoke in my cubicle, and he listened to all my foggy dreams and unrealized expectations. He held my hand without disturbing me and kept mentioning my strength enigmatically. While we communicated, he massaged my horrendously stiffened limbs, which the hospital should have been obliged to do following the nightmarish agony of the injections. He wasn't sanctimonious like most priests and he asked me worldly questions like if I had a girlfriend. I told him I fancied Bessie and we laughed. Then he became mystical again, and declared with a final flourish that, "you don't know who I am, but in thirty years time, you will thank me."

Medication had divorced me from the feelings of my own body by destroying the nervous system, which led to a natural neurosis about even my sexual identity. God saw His opportunity and introduced me to His special fiend, Neil. Neil was a retired psychiatric nurse who lived two doors away from Bish-

Bishopsthorpe, who Colin was guided by in the Golden Lion of a Thursday night. Sometimes to bail Colin out from Neil's incessant wittering, I would show up to feed an already spiritualized brain boosted by the love of 'Father to Son'. Neil seemed like a regular pensioner with heart condition, walking stick, cloth cap and glasses, but he was unusual (bordering on weird) with skinny purple lips and a hyperactive falsetto voice, like Hilda Ogden.

One late Thursday night while we waved Colin off, Neil stopped me and announced that I was "on a path where you can do nothing wrong". I took to his decree marvelously and it seemed I had friends to guide me in many directions. Moreover when he stated these magnificent and hypnotic words, his temple seemed to shine with another lucky gift.

It was not long before I discovered the real truth. I trusted Neil after his magical and inspirational prophecy, and occasionally we would take an impromptu drink in a café without Colin. I was right about the gift which he had received in his twenties, after being incarcerated in an asylum himself. However, he had been restored and went on to work in a psychiatric establishment, healing some people who had been so lifeless "that they would have been better off dead." Touché! I cast my furtive brow back to Great Yarmouth and his purple lips trumpeted, "sorry about Norwich" in perfect harmony. Surely he couldn't already know about my Fall from Grace without any hint of its exposure from my person?

One night in the Golden before Colin had dropped in, he presented me a few silly anagrams for me to arrange in my spare time. After solving the easy ones it struck me how they were filled with strong sexual innuendo, practically homosexual. For example, was it merely coincidence that T.S Eliot, of course translated as 'toilets'? Even when Colin arrived on the scene his lewd aspersions continued to throw a spell over me, suggesting, what?

It got me to reflect upon why every girl I had ever wanted had rejected me and set out to break my heart, preferring instead to go off with uneducated plasterer types and drug pushers. Why were the objects of my desires like Bess always unavailable, and was it my subconscious that was attracting me to women I couldn't have, to save me from the guillotine of more UEA-style, mental illness? Or was it simply a matter of my large bulk, putting off women who couldn't do without a walking macho man? When Bessie tilted her beautiful head with powerful assurance to tell me that she "didn't really know why I didn't feel like a man", my mind had reached overload. Was I a woman? Could that be a possibility that explained all my youthful dereliction? I had read somewhere that mental patients got ill because they could not find their true place in society. Had I become insane originally from the density of a psychologically misplaced love for June? Panic. My keen spiritual brain kept concentrating on 'Father to Son': 'And when she comes along, she could be breaking it'. That didn't help either, because 'she' could have been me.

I sought refuge from this backbreaking assault on my faith from my entourage of sainted trustees. All bar none were adamant that I was hiding behind my longstanding and nagging doubts about female rejection, to falsely jump to the conclusion that I must be gay. David abruptly spluttered that: "I know you. You would never go with a man." Bess for once unstrung her emotions and started to recklessly entitle Neil as "this character". She was also "sure" about my "erotic thoughts towards women". Rod balanced the argument by taking me aside and correctly arbitrating that "the two young girls don't think you're gay, and when I asked Ilona, she agreed that "gay sex repulses you". Amber with true hot-headed ambivalence angrily advanced that Neil would go to hell. The proper and non-distorted truth was completely defended by Andy who simply diagnosed that I was having doubts because I hadn't had a girlfriend for a long time.

However why had the stream of lovelies not to have come my way in my prime been so cruelly assaulted by fate? All my questions could have been sanely answered if the medication had allowed just one sexual hormone to thrive. Then I could have been assured of my sexuality in seconds. I determined to discuss whether I was coming or going with the architect of my prescription drug abuse.

Coogan was fair-minded enough to admit that the drugs (indeed all drugs) are "evil", but after my recent admission he wisely conjectured that I became a suicidal risk without medication. Fifteen-love. Suddenly that inner voice that had wished Bess had been with me at UEA, broke through Dr Coogan's inner self. With controlled anger it forcefully reminded me that I had "total choice over any sexual partner". There was a split-second silence where I conjured up Ilona's imploring compassion to not doubt myself. However, Neil seemed unavoidable and I met him shortly afterwards in a Sydenham backstreet I had strode down deliberately to avoid him. He proceeded to knock seven more bells of faith out of me when he announced that the hospital patient who ecstatically proclaimed I was Jesus, "had a gift for telling the Absolute Truth".

I was bouncing up and down like I was on God's rubber pulpit. I knew I wasn't anyone, particularly Jesus, and I confirmed so in Bessie's counseling boutique without a word of contradiction. She sympathetically found it "interesting" that I must have suffered every prearranged disaster in God's Time to atone for the problems of each and every living organism, and that to heal social wounds, I must redress traditional and historical prejudices by being a schizophrenic, gay, transvestite. These dumbfounding statistics seemed as unreal and as far off as my student nightmare, but they were really happening to me once more.

And when it wasn't Neil, it was another minister of the Lord, like the Muslim cleric, Naseem, who smashed any faith I had left in a God of Love, with more suggestive riddles. One Sunday morning while carting a load of shopping back to my pad, he froze me with anxiety, when he confirmed the Jesus Doctrine by announcing that, "I may not agree with you and you may not agree with me, but you are still here to fight prejudice". This distressing bombshell was typically confusing. Did it confirm that he as a believer and I as a liberal were politically opposed in our stance on homosexuality, and was he ordaining me as a gay man to undo prejudice? With my insight into apocalyptic fixations, it seemed entirely appropriate that Jesus and Muhammed may not agree. Could they not agree to disagree? If they can't shouldn't we? Shouldn't we conform to each other's choice, to the reasonable and sound ideology of the heart, to type. If man is hostile to freedom, he might surely only conform to his chains. I was facing these ghosts once more. Here was the red pulpit bashing out its swollen teachings. Then I recalled the truth of what Roddie had said about some priest; " I wonder what he does after his sermons? What does he do on Tuesdays? What does He do on Tuesdays I mused.

In the end Neil finally pulled down the curtain on my true heterosexual inclinations, when, after I had laughed his banal homosexual innuendo in the pub, I invited him innocently back for a coffee at my flat. It was a potentially fatal arrangement but I was so vulnerably uptight and magnetically drawn to the next dire prediction of my destiny. Like his God, he didn't fail me when immediately he suggested that I liked having something "long and thick in my hands". I envisaged a life of gay permissiveness, and uncharacteristic night-life, and all the hard work I had completed at the hostel and with Bess, being washed out by the utterly smothering tide of unalterable destiny. Finally I evicted him politely to the doorway, where he hugged me in my despairing jumble of apathy, and kissed my cheeks in gentle capriciousness. When I later told Gord', the authority on sex crimes that I didn't even remember what had happened after that, he assessed that I had been the victim of sexual abuse. Ditto David after some appealing.

I saw no way out of the trap now. I wondered whether Naseem's remark meant I would not have another proper girlfriend for thirty years. Was God so in fear of my natural sexual impulses and their involvement with insanity, that he needed Neil to inform me that any romantic association with Amber would be "playing with fire". Would it take "ages" before I got another girlfriend, as he propounded with ruthless credulity?

He connivingly trapped me forever by also stating I was "not definitely gay", which meant I must be bisexual, and still able therefore to tender normal sexual improprieties towards Junie, Liz, Bessie, Amber and Ilona. The romantic optimism and assumptions of 'Father to Son' were crushed, and the endless computations drove me to desperation, without the hint of a psychotic episode.

There was no way out. If I had tried a planned suicide bid, it would have materialized at university. In my present case there was no proper excuse to burn all the rescue admissions I had undertaken since I had moved to Bishopsthorpe, five years ago. According to Coogan I had "done it all myself" so it would have been a manifold shame if I were to exterminate the English hero I had found in the trunk of the old 'him'. However God had crushed every bone in my body I had fought for, and as Phil Collins concluded; all the things I thought were safe did seem to be gone. Certainly the future I had long held out for had gone.

The battle was lost and I took twelve Procyclidine tablets from a disused bottle stored on standby in the drugs cabinet. It was an unintentional attempt to kill myself (Dave said they usually are), but for the first time the course was not intervened with by delusional reckoning. However it was more than a cry for help as my friends related. Strangely, I recounted to Colin what I had the night before, not realizing that I was still in mortal danger in this early morning hour. Colin responded so seriously that there seemed to be tears in his eyes. It would have been touching had it not been so scary.

Dave had taken leave that weekend to visit his elderly mother, so I had to hastily arrange a lift from my father to the hospital, before we had time to absorb what I had done in the night. In the car we barely spoke, and soon we were trying to find a doctor, in the middle of Lewisham Hospital's manic A+E Department. Eventually on a busy ward I was led to a spare bed where a doctor performed some routine tests, before being bleeped somewhere else.

My feet lapped over the edge of the bed trembling. I wanted to live so much, but Neil's sentiments callously deadened the flame lethargically.

Ten minutes later I could see a young male doctor in a white coat flapping like a caped crusader, sprinting straight towards my temporary bed. With a massive bout of relief, he breathlessly announced that I had not taken sufficient quantities of the Procyclidine pills, and that I was indeed going to live. And here endeth the lesson. Amen!

EPITAPH

It could be fictional. Until I introduced myself, madness didn't exist. Now you have met the person, you have unraveled the schizophrenia: the needs of psychosis, the pain, the deepest strength to overcome, the lone fight, the war against God, and the freedom of 'haves' to make 'have nots' clearly see. I am not a Shakespearean tragedy, more, one of his characters he depicted to bring in light. I was a Pericles, and a Falstaff, a Banquo, and a Rozencrantz and Guildenstern. I described myself as a Shakespeare without a shred of sonnet, utopian pentameter, the chalk marginally impressing on the blackboard. But believe me, I am a Shakespeare: as fictional as the real one, but as real as any fragranced sentence, as silenced as the dusty old volume of his Complete Works.

What you have seen is me in essence. A man, true, with hang-ups about expressing it, but a man with that very same essence which saved him from those hang-ups when the lion roared at him with schizophrenia. Is it the same for everybody? I cannot say everyone can understand it now I have squealed. However, maybe some people with schizophrenia can use themselves to overcome themselves – or it, or them, or Him, or life. Stick it out and they may cure each other one day. I am sounding as barmy as my beloved Michelle who unarrogantly believes I am better than Him. Indeed some things are to be taken more seriously, more level-headedly, more forgivingly than Him, like one's self. Self-preservation is not selfishness.

The picture I have painted separates an autobiographer from its subject, a real person safe from a real psychosis. I can only dream that it is not too late to exhibit something that is not clever or pretentious, rather, a theatrical aside to his audience who may see with fair play, a comment with identity, meaning and an upside-down beauty. May it hang the wrong way up in the latest minimalist art establishment.

www.ingramcontent.com/pod-product-compliance
Lightning Source LLC
LaVergne TN
LVHW051827080426
835512LV00018B/2763